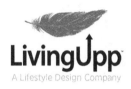

**LivingUpp**
A Lifestyle Design Company

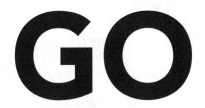

# GO

## ONE WOMAN. ONE VAN.
## A NEW BEGINNING.

**STACY FISHER**

Published by Intrinsic Publishing, a division of LivingUpp, LLC.

**www.LivingUpp.com**

Library of Congress Control Number: 2020923170

ISBNs: 978-0-9974853-6-3 (paperback);
978-0-9974853-7-0 (ebook)

# Contents

## PART III
### *Manifest*

# Preface

Whenever people hear that I—a forty-something, soon-to-be-divorced-for-the-second-time woman—made a solo trip across the U.S. in a Sprinter van, they usually have a few questions. While this book probably won't answer all of them, it will hopefully offer some insights about how I redesigned my life after everything fell apart.

My adventure led me through 20 states, spanned more than 10,000 miles, and gave me the space to grieve the loss of my marriage. But more than that, it helped me recover my sense of personal sovereignty.

Due to the circumstances that led up to the end of my marriage, I wrestled with how to best tell this story. For years, I've held onto secrets that I'm sharing for the first time openly in this book. And that's because, as is the case for most of our messy, life-changing experiences, there were other people involved in the unfolding of my story.

For that reason, I've chosen to omit names, change names, and leave out some specific details in order to honor the wishes of those who have been a part of my journey. (Plus, I've had the misfortune of having someone I trusted publish parts of my personal story in their book, and it felt awful.)

It's safe to say that we've all made choices that we later wished we hadn't. No one is perfect, and I believe that everything we experience in life has been carefully orchestrated for our highest good, even if it doesn't feel that way at the time.

If just one person feels empowered after reading this to lift themselves up out of the darkness, then it will be worth my discomfort. This trip was one of the greatest experiences of my life, and I hope that it offers you hope and encouragement if you happen to be facing a similar turning point in your life.

# Introduction

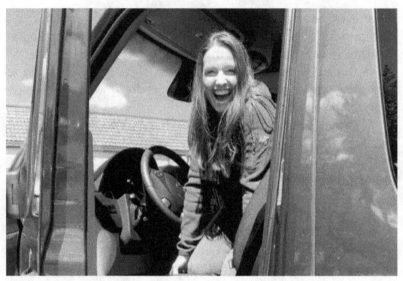

*Stacy in her Sprinter van (photo credit: Mitzi Cole)*

Buying a van, giving away the majority of my possessions, and setting out on a spontaneous drive across the country after my marriage fell apart wasn't in my original life plan—not even close. But then again, neither was being a twice-divorced, forty-something woman who had no clue what to do with her life. Looking back, that time in my life is now one of the greatest highlights.

But van life wasn't always glamorous. Most of the images you've probably seen on social media—the selfies of cute couples and their dogs with picturesque landscapes in the background—gloss over the reality of greasy hair, sweaty armpits, and van clutter. And it's hard to snap pictures when you're being harassed by a weirdo in the middle of the night.

While there were some challenging moments during that trip, it was liberating to feel untethered to the structured lifestyle that I clung to for most of my life. The life of a vagabond is vastly different from the civilized 9 to 5 lifestyle that most of us choose. Having freedom was wonderful, but not having roots also felt extremely unsettling at times.

With just 40 square feet of space to fill inside the van, to say that I downsized my life is putting it mildly. Placing childhood Christmas tree ornaments in the donation bin stirred some emotions for sure, but it felt really good to give new life to things that had mostly been relegated to the garage for years. I realized that I didn't need to hold onto things to preserve the memories attached to them, and I learned that the process of letting go was really more about choosing what to keep.

The early days of my cross-country road trip were some of the most difficult. I remember the strange mix of fear and excitement that I felt the day I left for my trip on the fourth of July.

But somewhere along the way, I started to feel like myself again—not the invisible, watered-down version of me that I'd allowed myself to become.

The road is where I recovered my independence, but the road isn't where my journey began.

# PART I:
## Survive

# Coffee and ~~Donuts~~ Divorce

We decided to end our marriage on a Sunday morning while drinking coffee on the living room couch. After just eight short years of marriage, it was time to come to terms with the truth that our efforts to repair the relationship had failed.

I took a few deep breaths and then a sip from my warm coffee mug, trying to prepare myself for the conversation that would ultimately determine the rest of my life.

My face was expressionless, my hair unbrushed. I was wrapped in my warm, fuzzy robe. It had become my only source of comfort, insulating me from the coldness that had slowly crept into my life over the past several years.

I felt queasy. I still didn't know what I might say when it was time to speak my truth. I'd known the man staring back at me for 33 years. We'd been high school sweethearts, prom dates with awkward wallet-sized photos to prove it. Then in college, like so many young loves, we went our separate ways, both marrying other people and moving on with our lives.

An unexpected twist of fate reunited us years later when a mutual friend emailed pictures of her new baby to a group of high school friends. I'd noticed his email address among them, so I sent him an innocuous message to ask, "Where has life taken you?"

But that email reopened the door to the possibility of more. And soon, it became apparent that the spark we thought we'd put out all those years ago had never quite been extinguished.

The universe seemed to be issuing us an invitation for a second chance at the fairytale. Except I was still married at the time.

After divorcing my first husband, I reunited with my high school sweetheart, and we eventually married. Things were wonderful at first. We traveled. We lived spontaneously. We laughed. We went on adventures. Life was great—until it wasn't.

When I discovered that he was having a relationship with a woman outside our marriage, it shattered me. I felt betrayed. I felt disregarded. I felt like a chump. But as devastating as it was, it seemed karmically appropriate, given that I'd had an affair during my first marriage as well.

While that fact gave me some perspective, it didn't do much to dull my heartbreak. Being the betrayer doesn't feel good either, but being betrayed is indescribably painful.

So, I retreated. I held onto my secret like it was a child that needed my protection. I only shared my reality with a few people close to me—just in case I needed a temporary place to stay if I ever decided to leave.

At first, I wasn't sure if I wanted to stay or go. I was in a state of shock, and stuck in survival mode. I trusted no one, and lived in a constant state of worry about what I might discover next. I was barely functional, and completely unable to consider any options for my future.

That's the same way I felt in that moment sitting on the couch. All week long I prepared myself for our meeting. I journaled. I spent time in meditation. I considered all the different scenarios that might surface during our discussion, and what I might do in response to each of them.

The decision to hold the fateful meeting came after an intense emotional eruption that made it impossible to deny any longer that our marriage was nearing its end. He had just returned home from a business trip, which was nothing unusual. I'd gotten used to him being away three or four days a week. But that night, I'd planned a special dinner. I set the table with beautiful Waterford china, crystal wine glasses, and linen napkins, and I'd corked a special bottle of wine that we'd picked up on an anniversary trip to Napa a few years earlier.

But the moment I sat down at the table, something came over me. Tears began flowing uncontrollably before I even knew what was happening. I couldn't catch my breath. It felt like a wave of knowing, or a deep realization. But whatever it was, it caused an intense surge of emotions that rendered me powerless. I could no longer suppress my unhappiness. And I didn't even try.

I pushed my chair back from the table and excused myself. Still sobbing, I climbed the stairs to the bedroom, shedding my clothes as I walked toward the shower. It was the only place I could think of to go. I turned on the faucet and waited for the steam to begin rising before stepping in and closing the door behind me. The hot water stung my face as it poured over my body, washing away the salty tears that had already started to feel sticky on my cheeks. I slowly eased myself onto the floor and let the water wash over the back of my neck. It offered some relief, but I knew it wouldn't be enough to fix what was broken. Soon, the entire room was filled with steam. I felt hidden. Invisible. Safe.

Unexpected emotional meltdowns had become a regular occurrence for me. I hated it. I hated that I wasn't able to keep my emotions in check the way I'd somehow managed to do in the past. At first, my outbursts had a positive payoff: his attention and affection. But as time went on, my suffering was met with little compassion, and I felt alone and disregarded. That had been my reality for the better part of two years.

Later that night, after I had finally calmed down enough to have a conversation, we both agreed that it was time to address the only question left to answer: Were we willing to stay and do more work to save the relationship, or was it time to go our separate ways? We'd hoped the week would give us enough time to fully consider the weighty decision at hand, without making a rash decision while emotions ran high.

As I stared back at the man sitting next to me on the couch, there was nothing familiar about him. Eyes that had once been so bright and full of life now appeared cold and distant, if not indifferent. The past few years had been painfully difficult for both of us. Broken marriage vows are never pretty.

I knew that the only possible way we could salvage the marriage would be if we both agreed to return to therapy. But if just one of us was unwilling, staying would no longer be an option.

And the truth was, we'd already done a lot of work. We'd already endured countless therapy sessions. We'd already read and discussed books on the topic of infidelity and boundaries. And we'd already invested time and energy into spending more quality time together. But usually, the latter only led to more arguments.

So, the question wasn't really *if* we had tried, but rather if we had tried hard enough.

My mind and heart were still at odds, but I knew that I couldn't go on living the way we had been. Besides, if *he* wasn't willing to invest anything more into the marriage, it wouldn't really matter where I stood.

After another sip of coffee and a deep breath, I mustered the courage to begin the conversation. "So, where are you on all of this?" I asked. It was a simple enough question, but a heavily loaded one.

My intuition already knew what he was going to say. In the darkness of the early morning, our sullen faces told the fateful story of finality before any words were spoken. We both looked tired. It was clear that change was inevitable, and my heart knew that our conversation that day would be the beginning of the end for a fairy tale that had never really existed. The law of impermanence was about to prove true, just as it always does.

As he began to speak, I immediately felt my stomach tighten. I braced myself for the blow that I was certain his words would deliver. No matter what he said, our lives were going to change forever.

Tears spilled down my cheeks as I listened to him share his doubts about the viability of our marriage. Even though I knew he was right, it was hard to hear that he wasn't able to give anything more to the relationship than he already had. I inhaled deeply. I didn't disagree, but I also knew the truth: It wasn't so much that we were un*able* to give anything more, it was that we were un*willing*.

Once we'd both had a chance to share our thoughts about our best path forward, the conversation shifted. It was no longer about whether to stay or go; it was about how to carefully untangle our lives so that we could each go our separate ways.

Then, without emotion, we calmly and pragmatically mapped out a plan that protected our mutual assets, minimized the discord between us during the transition, and accelerated the uncoupling process.

As sad as it was to face the thought of yet another divorce, I was grateful that we were at least able to maintain enough composure to focus on a mutually beneficial resolution. We both deserved to move on with our lives, and we deserved to do it peacefully.

Surprisingly, the final acknowledgment that our marriage had reached its end wasn't as difficult as I imagined it would be. In many ways, it was a relief. I'd been dancing back and forth between wanting to stay and wanting to go for years, and I suspected it had been the same for him.

Still, as much as I knew in my mind that parting ways was the right decision for both of us, it wasn't as easy for my heart.

Memories flooded my mind.

I thought back to our wedding day on Kauai, where we were surrounded by a small group of friends and family. The warm island breeze brought me back to 10:10 a.m. on 10/10/10, when we promised to love and honor and cherish one another for the rest of our lives. We lied.

I thought back to how constricting my wedding ring felt the moment I could no longer pretend our marriage wasn't failing, and how satisfying it felt to slip it off my finger and hurl it into the darkness.

I thought back to the day that my therapist said, "You'll remember it differently someday." I didn't believe her. But I did believe her when she told me that marriages that make it through infidelity are the strongest ones that exist. Or maybe I just wanted to believe her.

I thought back to the conversation he and I had in Paris just a few weeks earlier about possibly moving to Amsterdam for a few months. Now, we were mapping out separate futures with vastly different itineraries.

Our lives had been forever changed in an instant.

# *The Secret*

For years, I'd held onto hope that we would somehow find a way to make it through that difficult time in our marriage. I'd hoped that I would eventually find a way to trust him again, to recover my sense of self-worth, and to move beyond the heaviness that kept me feeling paralyzed.

But I also had moments of doubt. There were days when I couldn't imagine us being apart, and other days when I couldn't imagine us staying together another minute.

Part of the reason I stayed as long as I did was because I didn't want to look back and wonder if we would have been able to recover. Leaving the marriage at the first sign of trouble would have left me with lingering doubts about whether I'd made the right choice. And if I did leave, I wanted to be able to say that I'd given everything I could before throwing in the towel. But as time went on, my moments of doubt grew more frequent.

I remember one evening driving back from having dinner in downtown Seattle. We'd been arguing on the way home about something insignificant, like most of our arguments, and I'd finally mustered up the courage to say out loud that I wanted a divorce. But just as the words were about to leave my mouth, I remembered that it was his birthday. So I took a deep breath and, once again, held back my truth.

The next morning I'd lost my nerve to open the discussion to the possibility of going our separate ways and decided to give it more time.

But I was broken. There was no denying that. The tiny pieces of my shattered soul were no longer recognizable, even to me. I felt fragmented, unclear about my future, and unsure of what I even needed to feel whole again. But deep down I knew that I couldn't continue living the way I was living.

Between the demands of my corporate job and the emotional strain that I was experiencing at home, the stress had become more than I could handle. I found myself in a constant state of overfunctioning. My calendar was frequently double-booked, I wore my "busy badge" proudly, and I lived in a constant state of anxiety. I was in survival mode. Every morning I'd cake on makeup, hoping that no one at work would notice my puffy eyes, and the moment I sat down in my car at the end of the day, I'd break down in tears. Something had to give.

I knew that I had to let go of something, even if just temporarily, to give my body time to recover. After discussing it with my husband, we agreed that resigning from my job made sense, so I could get a handle on my stress levels and tend to my health.

So, on an early January morning in 2015, I pressed the send button to deliver my letter of resignation. Almost immediately, I felt a sense of relief. The tension in my body dissipated as I embraced the fact that I no longer had to wear a fake smile and pretend on a daily basis that everything was okay.

But there was also a small part of me that felt terrified. I'd just given up my only source of income and independence.

At first, I relished the quiet mornings at home. I had time to journal, prepare healthy meals, and exercise. I was free to use my time however I liked. But with the extra time on my hands, I found myself slowly sinking into a state of depression. I hadn't considered that my job had also served as a distraction, limiting the amount of time I had to feel sorry for myself. I knew that I needed something to occupy my time—but something with low levels of stress.

Not long after I submitted my resignation, I decided that I needed something positive to focus on, and that's when LivingUpp was born. I'd chosen the word upp, which initially stood for uniting people with positivity, because it's what I wanted so desperately for myself. I wanted to break free from the negative thoughts that kept me trapped in my suffering. I was tired of feeling broken, and I was ready to find the strength to pick myself back up again.

But over time, it evolved into *uniting people with possibilities*. Because life offers up infinite possibilities. We're the ones who create our own limits through our fears, beliefs, and choices.

Initially, LivingUpp was to be a simple blog, an outlet for my thoughts and a way for me to transform my grief into something more positive. Positivity was medicine. It lifted my spirits and kept me from spiraling into a pit of sadness.

But it still wasn't enough to occupy my time. I began perusing job postings, hoping that a part-time job would offer me a distraction without completely consuming my time and energy. When I noticed a listing for a temporary position at a local greenhouse, it seemed like it might be a good fit, so I drove over to fill out an application. A few days later they offered me the job.

Working at the greenhouse was perfect. It reminded me of my college job in a candle factory, where my days were consumed by straightforward, repetitive work. And the best part was that I didn't have to take my work home with me at the end of the day. It kept my mind busy, leaving me less time to swirl into a negative spin of rumination.

Being surrounded by beautiful flowers and plants all day was good for my soul. But soon the temporary position ended, and I was back to having too much time on my hands.

Because of the circumstances that led up to the end of my marriage, I didn't feel comfortable speaking openly about it. I worried that friends would try to convince me to leave the relationship. I worried that people who hadn't been through what I'd been through would judge me for staying. And I also worried that people would judge him for his behavior.

For that reason, I only divulged my secret to a handful of people who were close to me, mostly because I needed a sounding board, but also just in case I needed a place to stay for a while if things continued to deteriorate.

But each time I shared my secret, I felt worse. I didn't have the emotional bandwidth to answer the barrage of questions that almost always followed. *How did you find out? Did you know the other woman? Are you sure it's over between them?* Frankly, talking about the situation stirred up old emotions that I was tired of reliving over and over again.

And the truth is, I didn't want to shame my husband any more than he had been already. We'd been through the truth-telling process. We'd been to therapy. And we'd done what we could to rebuild the foundation of our relationship.

But as time went on, when it seemed appropriate, I began sharing my secret more openly. I spoke candidly with women when the topic of infidelity came up organically in conversations. I even shared my story from the stage a few times as a keynote speaker on the topic of self-care. Little by little, the heaviness of my secret didn't feel as heavy.

But, still, I had moments. Just when I thought I'd turn a corner on my healing, more feelings of anger and bitterness would creep back in. I wanted to believe that I was a woman who knew her worth, who was confident enough to walk away whenever she was disrespected. But it just wasn't as simple as I'd imagined.

I also struggled to answer a question that I would never be able to answer: *Why?*

*Why* had this happened? *Why* had it happened to us? *Why* had it happened to me? But I soon realized that it was a pointless, unanswerable question.

Because *why* anything?

But secrets are heavy. They require constant protection. They keep us prisoners, forcing us to wear masks in order to keep them hidden. My secret had grown so heavy that it wasn't only interfering with my healing, it was also interfering with my health.

I cried on a daily basis. I was drinking too much wine. I had no appetite. I wasn't sleeping well. And in the months preceding that conversation on the couch, I experienced a series of health issues, including bouts of heartburn (one of which landed me in the ER), skin rashes, insomnia, headaches, irregular periods, and nausea.

Months, if not years, of denying the magnitude of our broken relationship had taken more out of me than I realized.

# Hello, Self-Care

It was my therapist who first suggested that I focus on self-care. I was familiar with the term in a medical context. Self-care was a core component of diabetes care, and as a dietitian, it was something that I often addressed with patients. But I'd never considered the possibility that my own lack of self-care might have contributed to the physical symptoms I was experiencing.

My therapist also called attention to my lack of social support. In the two years since I'd moved from Austin to Washington State, I'd made little to no attempt to cultivate new friendships. My social circle was limited to my work colleagues, my husband, and a few long-distance friends who I was lucky to see in-person once a year, at best. I hadn't made room for anything that wasn't related to my job or my marriage.

When she asked me if I had anyone that I felt comfortable calling at 2:00 a.m. if I ever needed help, I couldn't think of anyone. And that was a scary realization. I had allowed my network to dwindle. My closest friends and relatives lived thousands of miles away, and it was the first time that I realized my husband was my sole source of support.

That's when self-care became my priority.

At the end of each of my appointments, my therapist had gotten into the habit of handing me a small piece of paper with a printed message on it. Some were messages of hope, some were reminders about my worth, and some offered words of encouragement.

But one message that still sticks in my mind today came as a giant wake-up call. The message went something like this: *If you aren't being treated with respect, check your price tag because maybe you marked yourself down.* And it was true. I had marked myself down. There was no doubt about that. I had deeply discounted myself, and I'd allowed others to do the same.

Over time, self-care became an undeniable necessity, and ultimately, it's what pulled me out of the darkness. It's what saved me.

The first area of my life that needed attention was my mindset. Bouts of negative thinking, along with reliving painful memories in my mind, left me feeling numb and trapped on a daily basis. In many ways, my pessimism became an addiction, and my victimhood became my identity. Except it was a secret identity.

The experience gave me a lot more compassion for those who struggle with alcohol and substance abuse. I could see how tempting it was to seek out anything to dull or numb the pain. Not feeling anything at all is easier than moving through the discomfort. But, in the end, moving through the discomfort is the only way to truly find relief.

Before discovering self-care, my default coping strategy was self-neglect. Ignoring my needs seemed fitting, considering that there was a part of me that didn't think I even deserved to feel good. I was punishing myself for putting myself in that position to begin with, and for keeping myself in it as long as I had.

It reminded me of the small apartment I'd rented just after divorcing my first husband. I'd been feeling the weight of my guilt over my affair, and I hadn't realized that I was punishing myself for it. The apartment was a small space in the basement of a house, and the rent was just $275/month. But I had to wear flip flops in the shower because the drain would constantly back up with a questionable substance that I preferred not to know the source of.

And I didn't recognize it as self-punishment until someone close to me pointed it out.

"When are you going to stop punishing yourself?" she'd asked.

All the subtle ways that I'd disallowed myself to experience joy reinforced my feelings of unworthiness to receive it. But I wanted more than anything to be able to feel good again.

My exploration of self-care began as a series of small experiments. First, I tried yoga, and my weekly Yin yoga class became something I looked forward to. Yoga offered a quiet space for me to momentarily let go of my sadness and reconnect with my body. All the tension and tightness became more obvious as I moved through the various poses and stretches.

Next, I delved into meditation. Jon Kabat-Zinn's book *Wherever You Go, There You Are* helped me understand that there's no such thing as a wrong way to meditate. I tried a few random guided meditations before falling in love with one that was narrated by Danielle LaPorte called "Creation Space." Meditation quickly became part of my morning practice, helping to make me feel grounded throughout the day.

Journaling had already been part of my daily routine since I was very young. As an introverted, only child, I often turned to my journal to process things that were happening in my life. Being able to unleash my thoughts—both positive and negative—onto the pages of my journal offered a safe space for me to release intense emotions in a healthy way.

And despite the fact that I'd been a dietitian for fifteen years at that point, my eating habits needed a makeover too. Indulging in wine and comfort foods had become an easy way to soothe my emotions. And while I'd only gained a few extra pounds, it was enough to take a toll on my health in the form of heartburn and unexplainable aches and pains. One night, I ended up in the ER with what I feared might be a cardiac event. Thankfully, it turned out to be nothing more than a bout of extremely painful gastric reflux. But it got my attention, nonetheless.

The ongoing stress, which I was certain had something to do with the fact that I'd been suppressing my secret, was beginning to threaten my health. I knew that I needed to change my day-to-day habits sooner rather than later.

And then I woke up in the middle of the night with a clear vision—it was of a circle with various interconnected pieces. I stumbled out of bed into the darkness and felt my way to my office, where I sketched out a sphere-like pie structure with various slices that depicted areas of my life that I needed to strengthen. Each of the 8 areas within the circle were unique, yet also dependent on the others for wholeness.

As I sat back and looked at the circular diagram, I knew that it was important, even if only to help me piece my own life back together. And that's when the first version of the 8-dimensional self-care framework was born.

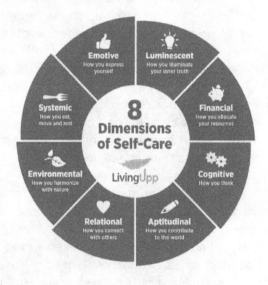

*The 8 Dimensions of Self-Care framework*

As I continued to explore self-care on a deeper level, I noticed that some self-care activities were more effective and enjoyable for me than others, and I realized that self-care is a very uniquely individual experience.

In an effort to expand my personal collection of self-care strategies even further, in 2016 I undertook a year-long self-care challenge. Every day of the 366-day leap year, I experimented with a new self-care activity. The objective was to gain a deeper understanding of which forms of self-care were most effective in supporting my well-being, and which were not worth my time or effort.

Many of the popular self-care rituals, such as taking spin classes, knitting (I'm a crochet girl), and attending social gatherings, weren't all that enjoyable to me. Over time, I learned that I preferred indoor symphonies over outdoor concerts, reading over binge-watching a TV series, and writing haikus over coloring. It showed me that self-care is personal, and that it requires ongoing experimentation with new things.

Similarly, some of the self-care activities that I expected to be complete flops became part of my daily practice. While journaling was something I'd already done for years, I learned that weaving in an element of gratitude journaling helped lift my mood dramatically. And as resistant to meditation as I was at first, it quickly became something I looked forward to.

I discovered that mocktails were a great replacement for my evening glass of wine, and I was surprised to learn that I enjoyed reiki, reflexology, and acupuncture. And who knew that a scalp massage could be so relaxing?

This self-care discovery process taught me that some of the most important acts of self-care would require me to build more skills. I needed to learn how to be more effective at asking for what I needed, at forgiving myself and others for being imperfect humans, and at setting and honoring my boundaries. Because boundaries are nothing if you don't honor them.

Surprisingly, a lot of my favorite forms of self-care were also the least expensive, and required only small amounts of time. For example, my homemade treadmill workstation—a simple tray that attached to the top of the treadmill rails—cost just $14 to make and turned out to be something I used on a daily basis. Since Seattle's rainy season made it difficult to get outside on the trails, it was the perfect solution.

Day by day, I was learning what I needed in order to feel whole and healthy again. And whether I realized it or not at the time, I was slowly building a supportive self-care foundation that was moving me out of survival mode and into my rightful place as the designer of my life.

As I thought more about self-care, it occurred to me that it was slowly lifting me out of the funk I'd been in for months. I was finding little things to look forward to each day, like my morning practice and a few drops of lavender essential oil in the shower. As time went on, I was starting to feel more like myself.

It became apparent that I needed a better system for identifying where to direct my limited energy, though, and I soon expanded the 8-dimensional model to include an assessment that helped me quickly identify my needs. I called it the "Rate Your 8 Self-Care Assessment," and I included it in the first edition of *The Self-Care Planner* and later, *The Lifestyle Design Planner*.

Every day, as part of my morning ritual, I'd rank each dimension of my life on a scale of 1 to 10 to determine where to focus my resources that day. That simple exercise continues to be part of my daily routine today.

But the mental, emotional, and physical aspects of my health weren't the only areas of my life that needed attention. In the three years between the realization that our marriage was in trouble and our conversation on the couch, I struggled a lot with my self-worth.

And because I hadn't invested much in building friendships, I felt more and more isolated as the strain on the marriage grew. But the idea of attending social events pushed all of my anxiety buttons. I dreaded the mere thought of having awkward conversations with strangers, so I opted to start a book club instead. I figured at least I'd meet some other introverted bookworms who could potentially become friends.

And because I got to choose the books for the book club, it also played a role in my healing process. We read books like Brené Brown's *The Gifts of Imperfection*, Will Bowen's *A Complaint Free World*, and Henry Cloud and John Townsend's *Boundaries*. I was desperately seeking anything that would ease my suffering and make me feel whole again.

# Champagne & Chickens

But after a few months, I realized that as much as I dreaded social gatherings, I still needed to expand my social network further. I learned about an event that had been recommended to me by a woman I'd met at an earlier event, so I decided to attend.

There, I found myself surrounded by a room filled with kind, energetic women who all had clearly invested in themselves. It was there that I met a wardrobe stylist named Lisa.

I was immediately drawn to her presence. She looked pulled together and professional, but also kind and approachable. I'd felt invisible for so long, and I was envious of her magnetism.

As far as my own wardrobe was concerned, my closet had slowly devolved into a black and white chameleon-like wardrobe. Plenty of people choose minimalist wardrobes like these on purpose, but I hadn't done it intentionally. It was something that happened almost without my noticing.

And to make matters worse, I didn't even feel good wearing my clothes. The bland wardrobe had simply become easier to manage, just one more way to conserve my dwindling energy levels. The only clear benefit was that it allowed me to stay invisible. By not calling attention to myself with my wardrobe, I could fly under the radar. No one would notice me, and that made it less likely that I'd have to answer any difficult questions, like "How is life?" My wardrobe offered a protective shield, making me unapproachable. But that also made building a support network even more challenging.

I was tired of hiding. I wanted to feel alive again, but I knew I needed help. A few weeks after we met, I hired Lisa to help me rebuild my wardrobe—and my sense of self.

First, we focused on determining my best colors. I'd already guessed that black and white weren't among them, and I was happy to learn that the colors she had selected as my best colors were also the ones I was naturally drawn to. I loved the earthy tones: deep greens, chocolaty browns, and creamy shades of beige.

Next, we identified my shape. I already knew that I was top heavy and short waisted, but beyond that I was clueless. Shopping for clothes wasn't something I enjoyed. The mere thought of how many hours I'd wasted trying on dreadful outfits nauseated me. After taking a few measurements, Lisa then proceeded to share some ideas about the types of clothing that would accentuate my assets and conceal my concerns. I was stunned by how a few simple adjustments could change everything.

Finally, we made our way to my actual closet, where she carefully sifted through the contents piece by piece. For each item that I tried on, we discussed how it made me feel—what I liked or didn't like about the color, shape, or style.

But when it came to defining my style, I drew a blank. I didn't think I had much of a style. As our conversation continued, and as I noticed which of the pieces of clothing were among my favorites, it became clear that I *did* have a style. It's just that I had chosen black and white instead.

Working with Lisa was some of the best money I ever spent on my personal development. I just never realized how important it was to understand how my colors, shape, and style played into my personal brand.

Our work together gave me a significant boost of confidence, and not only helped me remember who I am, but in many ways it gave me permission to show up more authentically—without feeling like I needed anyone's approval or permission to be myself.

Part of Lisa's package included a guided shopping trip, so as we worked our way through my closet, we simultaneously made a shopping list of things I might want to consider adding to my wardrobe.

When the shopping day arrived, I was so excited. I'd never had my own personal shopper. I thought it was something only rich people did.

At a local department store, Lisa pulled a brown suede jacket from a rack and said, "What do you think about this? It's very champagne and dirt!"

We both laughed at just how accurate the description was. Little did we know that phrase would eventually inspire my slightly modified personal brand: Champagne and Chickens.

# Forgiveness

Another woman that I was blessed to meet around the same time was a forgiveness coach named Brenda. We met at a networking event that I'd gone to reluctantly, and I was immediately drawn to her positive energy.

We later met for coffee, and it was during that conversation that I learned about patterns. I realized that my life had played out in some very recognizable patterns, and as I examined my life through a bigger lens, I saw it in six-year increments.

Almost every six years I moved to a different city, and there were some pretty clear patterns in my relationships as well. I had repeatedly chosen men with similar qualities, and it became more apparent why I had similar experiences within each of those relationships.

The more I worked with Brenda, the more I began to see that each of my life experiences—even the heartbreaking ones—had been designed with my highest good in mind. Through that new lens, life itself appeared to be a design project.

I began to see that the people who triggered the most intense emotions within me were some of my greatest teachers. They served as a mirror, reflecting back to me things I wasn't able to see on my own. And while it was difficult to accept at first, I realized that the things that upset me about them were really things that upset me about myself. Because the truth is, everyone we meet in life has something to teach us.

Through our work together, Brenda invited me to see my experiences differently. And it changed everything. All of it. Every detail of the experience. It transformed my suffering into some of my greatest lessons. It transformed my sadness into curiosity. And it transformed my bitterness into compassion.

Slowly, I regained my strength, self-confidence, and personal power. It became clear that forgiveness is a process—one that would take much more time to expose all the layers so I could take what I needed from it.

# A Cold Couch

When the memories finally faded, I realized that I was alone, sitting on the cold couch. I didn't remember him leaving. But I remembered the decision we'd just made. I felt numb. It was really happening. This was it.

I felt disappointed, but it was mostly disappointment in myself. It was becoming more apparent that my level of disappointment was directly proportional to my expectations. I felt embarrassed that I'd stayed in the relationship as long as I had, once again ignoring my intuition that it was time to go.

I struggled to understand why I hadn't respected myself more, why I hadn't had the courage to walk away sooner, when I still had a source of income and the strength to rebuild my life. I wondered why I hadn't been willing to acknowledge that our efforts to repair the marriage hadn't paid off the way we'd hoped.

But I knew the answer was that I wanted to be sure. I wanted to be able to say, when we finally reached the finish line, that I'd given it my all. And I had.

My thoughts returned to the cold couch beneath me. From the front window, the glow of the sunrise began to cast out shadows from their hiding places in the living room. The shadows had been much easier to ignore in the darkness. Just like the truth.

Suffering. That's what we'd been doing. We'd both accepted it for so long that it felt normal. So, the thought of replacing suffering with peace felt good. *Really* good. It gave me hope. I was ready to let go of the suffering.

My coffee had long since turned cold, but my fingers were still gripped tightly to the handle. I quickly shifted my mind to the logical, operational side of what we'd just decided to do. It was easier to focus on *doing* than to allow myself the luxury of *feeling*. I began to make mental lists of things I needed to complete to set the wheels of separation in motion.

In the days that followed our conversation on the couch, the numbness continued. It had to. Removing myself from the pain was my only hope for surviving the whirlwind of change that was coming. And it was coming whether I was ready or not. I did my best to prepare for the chaos that was inevitable. Uprooting my entire life was going to take every ounce of strength I had, and I had to keep moving forward. Grieving would have to wait.

I wavered between feeling excited about the possibilities for my future and the sadness over the life I was leaving behind. The sadness was more intense, its tentacles wrapping around me tightly, immobilizing me for long stretches of time. At random moments throughout the day, I'd lie in bed with tears streaming down my face, trying to understand how my life had come to this point. It was nothing like I'd imagined it. I wondered how on earth I was ever going to be able to rebuild my life from nothing.

Journaling helped some. It had always been an important part of my self-care practice, even before I classified it as self-care. Whenever I faced big decisions, my journal had always been a source of guidance. There, I could sort out my options, vent my feelings and emotions, and create a clear plan to move forward.

More often than not, my journal entries have helped me see the truth of what's happening in my life, especially when my thoughts and emotions do their best to deceive me.

Big questions about my future loomed heavily in the back of my mind: *Where will I live when the house sells? If I choose to leave Washington State, will my car make a cross-country trip? How long will it take to sell the house? How long will I have to move all my things out after the house sold? Where will I store my things in the interim? What will I be forced to leave behind?*

*Will I be able to afford health insurance? How will I support myself financially?*

But all of those questions would have to wait. I couldn't afford to spend time on anything that didn't involve preparing the house for market or filing for divorce. I didn't have the capacity to focus on anything other than closing up that chapter of my life.

So, I made lists. Lists gave me comfort. Being able to see everything that needed to be done all in one place relieved the extreme anxiety that I felt on most days. Life felt chaotic. I was barely holding on. But lists helped me keep it together. I made lists of everything—items that I wanted to take with me, items that needed to be sold or donated, and decisions that I still needed to make. Every time I thought of something that needed to be taken care of for the transition, it went on one of the lists.

List making also offered a distraction. When I was making lists, I wasn't feeling anything. It occupied my brain in a way that helped me escape from the overwhelming sadness that had been lingering since the conversation on the couch. With the exception of an occasional emotional meltdown that left me wailing on the floor in a state of exhaustion, I'd gotten really good at suppressing my emotions.

When I wasn't making lists, I was making phone calls. I broke the news of the divorce to my close family members. They were as supportive as they could be from thousands of miles away, but they were also worried about my well-being as I waded through the transition alone.

I also broke the news to close friends. Some were shocked, and some weren't as surprised as I imagined they'd be.

I made doctor's appointments. Not knowing if or when I would have access to health insurance again after the divorce, I scheduled preventive visits, refilled prescriptions, and updated my lab work to make sure I was up to date on everything.

Grieving was still on hold; it would have to come later.

Most of the work of preparing our home for the market fell to me, since my schedule was more flexible and I didn't have to travel. I met with the realtor. I touched up paint. I dug up the septic tank for inspection. I hauled loads of mulch and pea gravel uphill to the back yard. I cared for our dog, whose health had been steadily deteriorating. And I picked through four decades of belongings, separating them carefully into piles for us to sort through together at some point.

I also handled the process of filing the divorce documents. With both of us being in complete agreement about the division of our assets, and since we didn't have children, there was no need to consult with an attorney.

What kept me going was knowing that the sooner I completed each item on the to-do list, the sooner it would all be over.

There were moments throughout the day when I'd forget what was happening. I'd be out running an errand and think about what to make for dinner. And then it would dawn on me that I was only cooking for one. Tears would come without warning—in grocery stores, at doctor's offices, and even at the farmers' market. A single song could trigger a memory that would send me into an emotional tailspin.

But one day something shifted. While out running errands, I broke down in tears in the car. It was raining and I was sobbing hysterically, barely able to see through the windshield. And then I heard these words come out of my mouth:

"No matter what happens, everything's going to be okay."

And I stopped crying. I believed what I'd said. I believed that everything really was going to be okay—eventually. And in that moment, my heart opened. My soul felt supported. I realized that I had a choice about how I responded, even while I watched my life unraveling around me.

I was tired of crying. I wanted to feel alive again. I was tired of feeling sorry for myself. I wanted to stop living a life of victimhood, and start thinking about my future. I needed to shift my energy toward what was next for me, and what I wanted my life to look like when it finally belonged to me again.

One big decision had already been made, but I still had another big stay-or-go decision to make: stay in Seattle, or find a new place to call home?

I wavered.

Some days I'd wake up thinking about how much I loved the Pacific Northwest, how much its emerald green landscapes fed my soul, and how much I would miss it if I ever left. Its peaceful, rainy days offered me the opportunity to snuggle up in a fuzzy blanket and spend the day reading. Its endless hiking trails offered me an escape from reality, even if only temporarily. Two or three times a week, I'd take hour-long hikes in the middle of the day to release tension and anxiety.

But on other days, I felt paralyzed with sadness. Driving past one of our favorite restaurants was enough to bring on the tears. There were just too many painful memories there, and I wondered how I could ever feel good again if I stayed.

I also couldn't ignore the fact that Seattle winters are not for the faint of heart. I knew the dark, dreary days ahead would make my healing process more difficult, if not impossible. My soul longed for sunshine.

Even so, it wasn't only the emotional strain that concerned me. Seattle is an expensive city to live in, and with no stable source of income, I worried that I'd deplete my savings too quickly. Signing a long-term lease felt impulsive. I didn't want to be locked into anything, at least not in the next few months.

I'd also heard from friends in passing that apartments were hard to find, and the ones that were available were well beyond my budget. And the idea of having a roommate wasn't appealing at all. I needed space. I needed to go inward to grieve. And I needed to do that alone.

As I carefully weighed my options, the indecision only added to my stress. The longer I waffled between choices, the more tension built up in my body. My shoulders felt tight. I had headaches. And I felt myself slowly inching deeper into depression. It scared me, and I worried that spending a Seattle winter alone might make me slip even further.

In my heart I knew that I'd have to leave Seattle in order to rebuild my life, but I just didn't know where to go.

Back in 2017, my soon-to-be ex-husband and I purchased a Sprinter van together. My obsession with vans began on Pinterest, where I became mesmerized by people who took a basic shell of a van, and converted it into a beautiful tiny home. Most buildouts included miniature kitchens, beds, and some even had bathrooms and showers. Conversions were becoming more and more popular, especially among outdoor enthusiasts on the West Coast. And for good reason. Unlike RVs, which are bulky and pricey, vans are much smaller, making them easier to maneuver. And since the shorter model of the Sprinter van can fit into a regular parking space, it can easily double as a daily driver.

Our plan was to convert the van slowly. It would be a side project, something we could work on while also spending some quality time together. We planned to use it for extended off-grid camping trips and weekend getaways. Tent camping had become much less appealing as we settled into our forties. Chasing mischievous raccoons with a penchant for stealing shoes in the middle of the night was no longer as amusing as it had once been.

It was a project that ignited a lot of excitement within me. For months, I spent evenings and weekends creating Pinterest boards, Amazon wish lists, and fancy spreadsheets with grandiose ideas about possible layouts for the van's interior.

But there was one teensy weensy little problem: We couldn't agree on the design. He wanted tactical; I wanted cute. He wanted a gear hauler; I wanted a bistro on wheels.

My vision for the van included a clean, white interior with swanky crystal drawer pulls and lace curtains blowing in the wind when the doors were open. I envisioned us enjoying afternoon happy hours beneath a shade tree, while drinking wine from crystal stemware. In my mind, van camping opened up so many luxurious possibilities.

So the idea of slinging a couple of army green cots in the back, cramming a camp stove in a plastic tub, and calling it good, didn't quite align with my dreamy buildout.

Looking back, I can see that our inability—or perhaps unwillingness—to compromise on the design was just one of many clues that a split was imminent. It was becoming clearer that we wanted to experience our lives very differently.

As we carefully orchestrated the division of our assets, one of the biggest questions that remained was deciding who got to keep the van. The 4x4 model had been difficult to find. We'd waited months for it to be shipped from Germany, and we'd heard the wait for a new one was nearing 18 months at the time. But when I thought about the kind of traveling and camping that I wanted to do, I didn't see myself needing a 4x4. In no scenario would I deliberately place myself on a road, or in weather conditions that required four-wheel drive. So, for that reason alone, it made sense to me that he should keep the van.

But giving up the van also meant giving up my dream. I wanted to travel. I wanted to experience the freedom of exploring all the destinations that had lingered on my bucket list for years. I wanted to see the vastness of Yosemite National Park. I wanted to stand beneath the Sequoias and admire their beauty. I wanted to feel the extreme heat of the California desert. And I wanted to stand in awe overlooking the Grand Canyon. The van would allow me to do those things easily.

Deep down, I feared that if I gave up on my vision of owning a van then, I might never have the chance again. I've watched so many people save all the good stuff in life for later. They put their dreams off until retirement, only to realize they didn't have the finances or the health to live out their dreams when they finally got there. I wanted to experience what was on my Pinterest board, and it made me angry to think that only one of us would get to see it come to fruition.

# The Clipboard

To help us get the house ready for market, our realtor, Amanda, arrived on a Saturday afternoon to do a walk-through of the house with me. She wanted to take a closer look at the property to see what might need to be repaired, redecorated, or removed.

I was ready to get started. All I needed was a solid list to work from.

I greeted her at the front door with a clipboard clinging tightly in my hands. As we walked room to room, I took copious amounts of notes, which soon became my life's purpose. My to-do list included the following:

- Remove alcohol from the bar
- Paint the ceiling in the kitchen
- Remove the furniture from the front porch
- Clean the windows
- Clean out the gutters
- Remove all appliances from the kitchen counters
- Repaint the baseboard on the stairs
- Remove various pictures and décor from the walls
- Secure my jewelry and valuables
- Roll bath towels and place them in baskets
- Re-grout the bathtub
- Remove all rugs
- Mulch the front and back yard
- Haul in more pea gravel and tidy up the backyard patio area

And the list went on.

When she left, I swallowed back tears as I considered the amount of time it was going to take to get everything completed. But it would get done; it would have to. I would just have to take it one item at a time and keep moving on to the next until it was done.

I was grateful that I had client appointments on my calendar. It offered a distraction from the chaos, and gave me something positive to focus on. But when I wasn't coaching clients, I was crossing items off my to-do list.

I couldn't stop thinking about the van. It weighed on my mind constantly, and I envisioned what it would be like to make a cross-country trip alone. I wondered how easy it would be to find internet access. If I became a digital nomad for any length of time, I'd have to figure out how to ensure that my clients didn't experience any disruptions. There were so many things to consider if I did end up choosing to spend a significant amount of time on the road.

When I wasn't dreaming about the van, I was hauling mulch and gravel, moving furniture, and contorting my body in strange ways in an attempt to paint the kitchen ceiling, something I'd put off since the kitchen remodel three years earlier.

# *Zoey*

And then another goodbye came without warning. By then, I'd gotten really good at them. I'd already said goodbye to my marriage, and I had just started coming to terms with saying goodbye to my home. But I wasn't at all prepared to say goodbye to my miniature dachshund, Zoey, who had become my only companion in recent weeks.

For years, she'd suffered a myriad of health issues, from seizures to back problems. But somehow, she always managed to pull through. In recent weeks, though, her flare ups had become more frequent. She was already taking more medication than most seniors I knew, and I often wondered if she could sense that big changes were coming.

Seeing her immobilized and in pain was more than I could bear, and it was clear that it was time to say goodbye. After a quick call to my husband to make the final decision, I made the arrangements to ease her suffering. When the veterinarian from Lap of Love arrived, I led her to Zoey, who was resting peacefully on her favorite bed in the kitchen. Like me, she loved feeling warm. When she wasn't outside, she was almost always curled up in one of her many blankets strategically placed throughout the house.

We sat down on the floor and turned our attention to Zoey. The vet asked me about her favorite toys, what she was like when she felt good, and helped me recall the beautiful moments I'd spent with her. We then discussed her deteriorating health while the vet did an assessment. It was clear that she was in pain, and even hospice care wouldn't be able to extend the quality of her life.

It was time to say goodbye.

I couldn't blame her for not wanting to come along with me on my next adventure. I still had doubts of my own. There were moments when I questioned whether I had the strength to start over again. So, while her departure was unexpected, it wasn't exactly surprising.

But her absence also created another void. For the past few weeks, it had been just the two of us. Aside from a few clanging dishes in the kitchen here and there, the tag that hung from her collar was the only audible noise in the house.

Just a few minutes later, that same collar hung from a hook near the sliding glass door. I didn't remember putting it there. I didn't remember saying goodbye. I didn't remember much of anything that happened that day. I'd have to mourn Zoey's loss later. I was running out of time and I still didn't have a place to live.

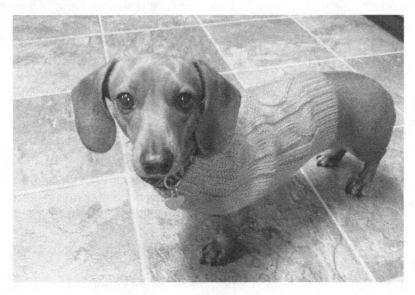

*Zoey*

# The Stage

In the midst of all the chaos, I was doing my best to continue running my business. While LivingUpp started out as a blog, in the weeks that led up to our conversation on the couch, I'd also launched a new coaching program, and several clients had already enrolled. This was yet another consideration I had to make as I thought about my options for relocating after the sale of the house.

Several weeks before my to-do list became consumed by the divorce, I had agreed to speak at a women's conference on the topic of self-care—except the message I had originally planned to deliver no longer felt truthful or relevant. I'd planned to speak about how vital self-care is in a marriage, especially ones that are facing insurmountable odds. And while that is indeed true, it felt inauthentic. Hiding the fact that my marriage had ended felt disingenuous. I wanted the message to be one of hope and of healing, but so much had changed.

Only two weeks had passed since we'd decided to separate, and now I had to figure out how to muster the strength to face a room full of women who were looking for inspiration. I scanned my closet and settled on one of my favorite green dresses. It's one that my wardrobe stylist, Lisa, had picked out for me, and it made me feel beautiful and powerful. I then painted my face with as much makeup as it could possibly hold, and hoped that it hid the dark circles and puffiness around my eyes.

When I arrived at the venue, the hotel lobby was already buzzing with voices. A few familiar faces greeted me with a smile, and the positive energy lifted my spirits. I found the table that had been set aside for me just outside the doors to the conference room. It was covered with a simple black tablecloth, and it was just big enough to display a few of the planners that I hoped to sell between breakout sessions.

I recognized a few women from other networking events I'd attended, some of whom I'd gotten to know well enough to share my secret. Knowing that I had friends in the room brought me a great deal of comfort, especially given my recent change in life circumstances.

Guests slowly made their way inside the doors to the conference room, where round tables with white linens awaited them. As they took their seats, my heart started beating faster.

The organizer of the event gave an introduction and overview of the speakers on the agenda. I felt humbled to be among them.

When it was my turn to speak, I was still unsure exactly how to weave my recent life changes into the presentation. I could choose to keep it a secret and deliver my original message. But that felt dishonest. Or I could keep it real and be honest about the fact that I was standing there before them in the middle of a crisis, barely functional, and in survival mode.

After the host introduced me, I climbed the small metal staircase at the end of the stage and took a few deep breaths. I knew in that moment that it would be best to allow my heart to do the speaking.

When I reached the podium, I looked down at my notes and then back at the audience. I don't know if it was the expression on my face, or if I'd been standing there in silence longer than I realized, but the room was silent. All eyes were on me. I took a few more deep breaths and started to speak.

"A week ago, today," I began, "my husband and I decided to end our marriage."

My heart raced as I processed what I'd just said out loud. I quickly looked back down at my notes for a moment before looking back up at the audience. I felt the weight of every eye in the room. I blinked back the tears that I could feel welling up in my eyes, and continued.

It was clear by the expression on many of the faces looking back at me that I wasn't the only woman in the room who had been in that place—that in-between place. It was a place of uncertainty, a place of quiet suffering.

Their faces carried a mixture of love, empathy, and compassion that gave me the strength to keep sharing from my heart. I went on to share that just days before, my life had been completely uprooted, that I was unsure what the future held for me. But the one thing I knew for sure was that self-care is a powerful tool that is also a source of strength and hope.

After I delivered the closing remarks of my presentation, I felt lighter. Being honest was the right call. I hoped my message hadn't been too heavy, and I hoped that it offered some hope to those who may also be facing unknown futures as well.

And then it was clear to me that it had.

Afterward, a woman approached me outside the conference room at my table with tears in her eyes. She extended her hand and grabbed ahold of mine, squeezing it gently.

"I've been where you are," she said. "And it does get better." She squeezed my hand again, and I thanked her for her words of encouragement.

And then another woman approached me. "I really appreciate that you shared your story today. I'm going through a divorce right now, too, and it's reassuring to know that I'm not alone," she said.

I was surprised by the number of women who stopped by my table to either share kind words of hope, or to say that my story was also their story. Our shared struggles had united us.

When I returned to my car, I felt physically exhausted but spiritually full.

# The White Whale

With the conference checked off my to do list, I was able to refocus my energy on the move. While I still hadn't completely decided on buying a van of my own, it sounded more and more appealing as time went on. I dreamed about it constantly, envisioning what it might be like to be untethered and free to wander the country. It was the only thing about my future that excited me.

Van life had become so popular that enthusiasts even had their own hashtag: #vanlife. Instagram, YouTube, and Pinterest had blown up in recent years with images of people all over the world living out nomadic adventures.

From a practical standpoint, I couldn't ignore the fact that it was the perfect time to consider the possibility of exploring a digital nomad lifestyle. I didn't have a traditional 9 to 5 job. I didn't have any children. I hoped to end up with a little bit of money in my savings account after the sale of our home. And I was in good health. But, perhaps more importantly, I didn't know if I'd ever have an opportunity like this again.

With the house being so close to going on the market, and with the paperwork for the divorce almost ready to be filed at the courthouse, I had to make a decision about where I was going to live when the house sold.

As I held the thought of buying a van in the back of my mind, I briefly considered some other equally bold possibilities, like taking an international job, or embarking on a solo backpacking trip around the globe, but both options felt more risky and extreme than I felt comfortable with. Suddenly, the van adventure didn't sound as outrageous.

Time and time again, my mind kept wandering back to the van.

Before we'd purchased the first van, I'd become obsessed with tiny homes. I'd watch HGTV shows that featured tiny homes. I'd created a Pinterest board that was filled with images of tiny homes. Many times, I'd envision what it might be like to downsize my life to the bare essentials, and actually live in a tiny home.

I relished the thought of owning less stuff. I wanted to spend more time living. I wanted to spend more time doing the things I loved, and less time doing things like dusting and reorganizing.

The idea of making a solo road trip felt strangely empowering. When I was six, my mom loaded up our Ford Granada and moved us to Florida. I remember lying on stacks of suitcases in the back seat, where I occupied myself with coloring books and crayons for nearly a thousand miles. It didn't seem like a big deal then, but perhaps that experience proved to me that major life transitions weren't that uncommon. Maybe there was a way to be adventurous without being irresponsible.

But the ultimate decision to move forward with buying a van and leaving Seattle came down to a series of simple math equations.

First, my car needed to be replaced no matter what. Since we'd already decided that he would leave with the new van, it made sense that I also leave with a new vehicle. But that wasn't the only reason I needed to replace my car. Because I was self-employed and without a consistent source of income, I also worried that I might not be able to secure a loan on my own if I waited until after the divorce. As I considered the options for replacing my car, I was shocked to learn that most SUVs were near or above the $50k mark, so about the same price as a van.

Second, there was the issue of moving expenses. When I found out it was going to cost $7k+ to ship a small POD filled with trinkets across the country, I laughed into the phone receiver. *Seriously? No, wait. You're being serious, aren't you?* That was money I would never ever, ever, ever be able to get back.

Third, I wasn't even sure where I wanted to live yet, and without a clear delivery destination, I'd be forced to pay a monthly storage fee. The idea of downsizing sounded more and more appealing, and I realized that it would be cheaper to replace items later once I decided where to replant my roots. Besides, a van was basically a moving truck on wheels, and I could at least sell it later if I ever wanted or needed to.

And because I wasn't sure where I wanted to live, the van also offered me temporary housing. While it was less than ideal from a comfort standpoint, it was essentially rent-free. I had no plans to become a full-time van dweller, but it did give me comfort to know that I wouldn't have to sign a long-term rental lease or impose on friends and family while I figured out where to relocate.

But perhaps the most important consideration was that the van provided what I needed the most. It bought me time. In the midst of all the chaos, I'd found it nearly impossible to make any decisions. I felt numb. I felt directionless. And making any long-term decisions seemed like a recipe for disaster. Keeping my options open for a while seemed like a smart idea. The van would give me a place to decompress and immerse myself in self-care while I figured out what to do next. I needed to feel grounded again before I made any important decisions.

And I still needed to grieve.

As I considered the drawbacks to van life, only two things came to mind. One was that the high roof would make it impossible to park in parking garages. That meant I'd have to find alternative parking options at hotels, airports, and shopping centers. The other drawback was that I wouldn't be able to go through drive-thrus, but that wasn't as much of an issue since fast food was a rarity for me. In general, they were both minor sacrifices; the benefits far outweighed the inconveniences.

As far as I could tell, the van made the most practical sense of all my options. It reduced the cost and complication of moving. It offered me a temporary housing solution. And it bought me extra time and space to figure everything out before deciding what I wanted to do next.

The van simplified everything.

While I was 99% certain that I wanted to move forward with buying a van, I still had some lingering doubts, mostly because it wasn't exactly conventional. I recognized that I was under a lot of stress, and I worried that my decision making might be clouded. With that in mind, I turned to a few close family members and friends to get some input. I wanted to hear how crazy my idea sounded to people who weren't living in emotional chaos.

Some were in full support of my dream, saying they wished they could do something similar. But others weren't as encouraging as I'd hoped. I heard reactions like, "Don't you think you should focus on getting a job?" and "Wouldn't getting a small apartment make more sense?" Their play-it-safe feedback made logical sense, but it was clearly rooted in fear.

I knew they were only concerned about my safety and well-being, but each comment carried a small vote of no confidence. It hurt to know that not everyone believed in me. In my already-fragile emotional state, I didn't need to be reminded that my life was a mess and that I'd eventually have to clean up that mess. But I also knew that, while it was a critical turning point in my life, it was also an amazing opportunity to create some joy in the midst of all the turmoil.

I already knew deep down what I wanted to do, and the truth was, I didn't really need or want anyone's input or permission.

If anything, in the back of my mind, I worried that if I didn't move forward with buying a van, I might end up regretting it for the rest of my life. I was terrified of looking back on that moment and feeling disappointed that I didn't have the guts to just go for it. And there would be no one to blame for the missed opportunity but me.

The truth is life is short—way too short to live a shitty one. Many people spend their entire lives in jobs they hate, squirrelling away acorns for retirement, only to discover that when they finally get there the promise of the good life was all a lie. They save all the good stuff for later, but when later finally arrives, either the money they were expecting isn't there, or they're in such poor health that they can't enjoy it. There's just no guarantee.

And the truth is, our dreams don't just show up on our doorsteps unannounced. They don't randomly bump into us in line waiting for a Caramel Macchiato at Starbucks. We have to make complicated and uncomfortable decisions to bring our desires to life. We have to find creative solutions to our problems. We have to relentlessly pursue our goals.

I wasn't ready to let go of my dream so easily. I wanted my own damn van.

Making the decision to begin searching for a van was a huge relief. It was one less decision that I'd have to make, so it freed up my energy to focus on squaring away the other pieces of my life.

I imagined myself on the open road, exploring possible new places to settle down. Even in my mind, it felt liberating and exciting to no longer be bound by normal day-to-day routines. It was an escape I desperately needed.

As I searched the web for popular tourist destinations, I started to consider all the places I might want to visit. Since it was early spring, the weather would soon be nice enough to go just about anywhere. By the time I'd be ready to hit the road, the snow would mostly be melted on the mountain passes, which would open up even more possibilities. My options were endless.

I thought it made sense to first check in with the salesman we'd purchased the first van from, in case there was something already there on the lot. I sent a quick email and learned that there was one white crew model available. I emailed him back immediately, saying that I would be down within the hour to look at it.

On the drive to the dealership, I felt elated. The thought of taking the plunge into van life gave me something to be excited about for the first time since my life had collapsed. The thought of living in a van was both crazy and sensible at the same time, just like me.

But when I arrived, my heart sank. The salesman was standing out on the lot showing the white van to someone else. My heart raced. Not wanting to be rude, I stood outside the front doors to the dealership, staring down at them. I thought briefly that the salesman might see me, and invite me down to join the conversation since he knew I was coming. But instead I squirmed impatiently as I silently prayed that it wouldn't be sold before I had the chance to snag it. I was feeling even more ready to commit.

Then I got an odd feeling in the pit of my stomach when I watched the two of them shake hands and part ways. The salesman looked up at me and began walking my way. My fears were confirmed when he broke the news that the van had just been sold. I'd watched the whole thing. I'd been ten minutes too late.

I was crushed.

A complete stranger had just ripped my dream right out of my hands, and I couldn't do anything about it. I blinked back tears, like I'd done so many times in recent weeks, and thanked him for his time. I could feel the emotional tsunami coming.

He chuckled, pointing to a smurf-colored blue van parked at the far end of the lot.

"This one's still available," he said with a smile. Clearly, it had been there for a while.

"Um, thanks, but I think I'll pass on that one," I said. I may have been desperate, but I wasn't that desperate. It just wasn't my style. While I was indeed nearing the point of desperation, I wasn't about to settle just yet. My search had only just begun.

When I got back to the safety of my car, I lost it. Tears rolled down my cheeks, and the sounds that came out of me were animalistic. I wailed like a toddler whose favorite toy had just been taken away. In a matter of minutes, I'd lost my white whale. But more than that, I'd lost the thrill of the adventure I'd been carrying in my mind.

The idea of buying a van had first been just a practical solution for the interim. It solved my immediate problems and made good financial sense. But as time went on, I became obsessed with the thought of being a "van girl." The van would be more than just a replacement vehicle; it would be my ride to the other side of the chaos.

On the drive home, I weighed the heaviness of my reality. The house was scheduled to go on the market in just three days, and our realtor expected it to sell immediately. The housing market in Seattle at the time was booming. There was very little inventory, which meant homes were being snatched up almost as soon as they hit the market. Bidding wars were common, and many homes were selling for over asking price.

Walking away with extra money in my savings account sounded nice, but a quick sale would also mean that I'd have less time for the actual move. I'd be lucky to have 30 days before closing once it sold. Four weeks isn't a lot of time to sift through 41 years of stuff, much less find a place to put it.

The truth was, I didn't have another plan to fall back on, and I questioned whether I even had the energy to create a new strategy. The pressure of the divorce, Zoey's passing, and the sale of our home had become too much. My head was spinning, and I felt exhausted.

About halfway home, I felt the urge to call my husband. We were still technically married, after all. I didn't have anyone else. We'd always made big decisions together, and even though we were separated, we still shared a lot of history. I dialed his number and held my breath.

When he answered the phone, I relayed what had just happened at the dealership and asked for his help with talking through my options. Thankfully, he was willing to help me explore some alternatives.

As we ran through a few ideas, like buying an SUV or keeping my current car and delaying the buying decision until later, I was starting to come to terms with the possibility that maybe the van wasn't meant to be. Maybe losing the white van was a sign from God or the universe that I wasn't supposed to go that route at all.

But the moment I heard myself say it out loud—that maybe a safe, conventional SUV was a more logical choice—it nauseated me. My dream hadn't included an SUV. Not in any scenario.

When we hung up the phone, I still wasn't clear about what I should do, but it felt good to at least have an outlet to vent my frustrations. I realized that I was going to have to get used to making big decisions on my own.

When I returned home, I spent the remainder of the day holed up in my office scrolling through the inventory of Sprinter vans at nearby dealerships, but none of the vans I found met my criteria.

Mercedes makes three models of vans: cargo, crew, and passenger.

Cargo vans are designed specifically for commercial use. They are built for couriers, delivery drivers, and contractors who need room to haul equipment and supplies. With no extra seating in the back and no windows on either side, it's the bare bones model. While it's cheaper than the other two models, it has a few drawbacks. For one thing, I'd have to eventually install windows, and that would be another expense. Some people might like the added security of not having windows, but I wanted to have at least a little natural light. And the other detractor was that cargo vans are classified as commercial vehicles rather than passenger vans. And from everything I'd learned in my research over the past year, that could pose a challenge later on, for a number of reasons.

Passenger vans are exactly what you might expect—built specifically to carry passengers. With three rows of bench seats in the back, the passenger van can carry up to nine passengers, not including the two front seats. But in order to have room for all my things, I'd have to chuck out the seats. The passenger van also has large windows that extend down both sides of the van. While I liked the idea of having the extra natural light, it didn't offer much in the way of privacy. In addition, passenger vans are more expensive than the other models.

The crew model was the sweet spot—and also why it was the most difficult model to find. It was perfect for people like me who eventually wanted to convert it into a campervan. With just one removable bench seat, it offered a lot of cargo space but was still classified as a passenger van. And with just half the windows of the passenger van, it offered the right combination of natural light and privacy.

But I was hitting a wall. Finding no vans that met my criteria in the area, I expanded my search to statewide dealerships.

Still nothing. Then, I extended my search to neighboring states. Nothing. After a few hours of scrolling and clicking, I felt defeated. I thought back to the blue van for a brief moment. *Nah.*

Wiping back tears from the intermittent bouts of sobbing, I found myself wishing that I could hug my sweet little dog, Zoey, who'd only been gone a week. I missed her. She always managed to comfort me during my emotional meltdowns, which had become more frequent in recent weeks.

With puffy lips and swollen eyes, I fell onto my bed and sunk my head into my pillow, releasing my fate to the universe. I had nothing left to give, and nothing to look forward to.

# Tenorite

The next morning, I woke up feeling calm and more rested than I had in days. Perhaps I'd been more exhausted than I realized the day before. I immediately felt a renewed commitment to the idea of buying a van, and I was determined to figure out how to manifest it.

After pouring myself a cup of coffee, I returned to my office and doubled down on the van search with a fresh set of eyes. By that point, I was willing to drive a couple hundred miles if I happened to find the right van. Heck, I even considered flying to another state if that's what it took. While the latter scenario wasn't optimal, and would only add another layer of complexity to my already-frenzied life, I held the option in the back of my mind, just in case.

A few minutes later, I came across an image of a dark gray crew van. I stopped scrolling. I took a sip of coffee from my mug and clicked the additional images on the page. The color was described as Tenorite Grey, just ever-so-slightly different from the Graphite Grey van we'd purchased together.

I scrolled through the images again and again, envisioning myself behind the wheel with all of my worldly possessions stowed neatly in the back.

*Free.*

I scanned down the page and noticed that the van was at a dealership in Lynnwood, just a few miles away from me. I stopped scrolling. *How had I missed it yesterday?*

It was the one.

I knew it was the one.

I immediately grabbed my phone and dialed the number to the dealership. My heart pounded in my chest, just as it had the day I watched my white whale swim away. When the receptionist answered, I asked to speak with someone in the Sprinter van sales department. The line clicked, and I was greeted by a voice recording.

I left a short message and hung up the phone. But my heart was still racing. I sat in silence staring at my computer screen. *What if he's talking to someone else about it right now? What if someone else steals this dream from me, too? How often does he check his messages?*

I'd already lost one van, and it felt too risky to wait on a return call, so I grabbed my keys, jumped in the car, and headed toward the dealership. At least I'd know immediately if it was even still available. If it wasn't, I could turn my attention back to the search.

I pulled into the dealership parking lot and found an open spot. The receptionist at the front desk of the lobby greeted me with a smile and informed me that the salesman was with another customer. My stomach tightened.

She directed me toward the waiting area, where I slid down into a plush leather chair, hoping that this wouldn't end as another missed opportunity.

Soon, I looked up and noticed a man wearing a wide smile walking toward me.

"Are you Stacy?" he asked.

"Yes," I said, standing up from my chair.

"My name's Lance. I hear you're interested in a Sprinter van," he said, extending his hand.

I shook his hand firmly, hoping that I didn't appear too frazzled or anxious. I wanted the van, but I also wanted a good deal.

After I explained that I'd seen the gray van on their website, he broke the news to me that the van wasn't physically on the lot yet.

"Right now, it's on a train somewhere in the middle of the country," he said. "But we expect it to arrive in a few weeks."

*A few weeks?*

I didn't have a few weeks.

With no guaranteed arrival date, and no way to track its current location, I'd be left to the mercy of the universe if I took the chance and bought it sight unseen. My mind swirled with what-if scenarios: *What if I bought it, but it didn't arrive before closing? What if it didn't arrive at all? And where would I store my things in the interim if there was a delay?*

It was decision time. Either I'd have to take the chance and hope that the van would arrive before the closing date on the house, or take a pass and continue my search.

"What do I need to do today to make sure the van is mine?" I asked.

"All I need is a $2,000 down payment, and I'll call you when it comes in." he said.

Thankfully, I'd thought to bring my checkbook along, just in case.

"Who shall I make the check out to?" I asked.

His face perked up. "Let's walk up to my office," he said, pointing to the nearby elevators that were just a few steps away from where we were standing. We stepped in and he pressed a button.

"You're really going to love it," he said. "They're great vehicles."

"I know," I said. "I already have one at home." He tilted his head and looked at me with a puzzled grin.

"My husband and I bought one last year and now I want one of my own," I said, shrugging. I didn't feel the need to share any more details about my situation. Frankly, I didn't have the energy to answer any follow-up questions. I knew that I wouldn't have answers for any of them anyway.

The elevators opened and I followed him down the hallway toward his office. He invited me to have a seat, but I was too amped up. I grabbed the checkbook from my purse and leaned over the desk to write the check.

Before the ink was dry on my signature, I tore the check from the pad and handed it Lance, thanking him for making the process so easy.

When I returned to my car, I melted into the driver's seat, both relieved and terrified at the same time. I was officially a van girl.

*What in the actual hell had I just done?*

I drove home in silence, my mind buzzing from the giant leap I'd just taken. It was official. I was going to have a van of my very own. And I was just going to have to trust that the timing would all work out the way it was supposed to. I didn't really have another choice.

It would either arrive on time, or it wouldn't.

# The Courthouse

The next day, I blinked back tears as I pulled into an open parking space at the county clerk's office. Next to me on the passenger seat was a manilla folder that contained a stack of signed documents, everything required to file a petition for divorce.

I'd spent the last couple of weeks researching the divorce process in Washington State. Because we didn't have children, and because we'd already come to an agreement about the division of our assets, it seemed like a fairly straightforward process. And since my schedule was more flexible, I volunteered to handle the filing process with the court.

Clutching the file folder tightly in my hands, I climbed the stairs to the courthouse. After moving through the security line, I found the elevator and headed up to the county clerk's office, where I took my place in line.

In front of me, there was a man holding a brown leather briefcase, fidgeting back and forth. In front of him, two women stood holding file folders. They both wore name badges that were attached to lanyards hanging around their necks. They were chatting quietly, laughing, and shaking their heads.

And then there was me, a scattered, middle-aged woman who had no fucking clue what she was going to do with her life.

Finally, it was my turn.

"Next," I heard a woman's voice say.

I stepped forward to the window, where the woman greeted me with a smile. I opened my folder and handed her the documents inside, hoping I hadn't missed anything.

"I wish everyone who came through here was this organized," she said.

I smiled. I'd spent more than a week combing through online resources before I found what I'd hoped were the right documents to file for divorce.

She turned back to her computer, tapping wildly at the buttons on her keyboard, and a few moments later, she stamped a date on the front page of one of the documents and handed it back to me.

"Next," she shouted.

The divorce was in motion; there was no turning back.

# *For Sale*

The next morning, a white FOR SALE sign swayed like a ghost at the end of the driveaway. Life as I'd known it for six years was coming to an end, whether I was ready or not.

When we'd bought the house six years earlier, I fell in love with the exterior immediately. The house was situated on nearly an acre of land with dozens of towering western red cedars and Douglas firs; flowering shrubs, like rhododendrons and azaleas; and endless tiered perennials that were wedged between stacked natural stone.

There wasn't a blade of grass to mow on the property. I giggled to myself remembering that we'd traded our lawnmower for a case of wine not long after we moved in. Not having to mow grass was an unexpected gift.

The interior of the house was a different story, though. Built in 1972, it was seriously outdated, with dark green carpeting, flowery pink wallpaper, and dark brown kitchen cabinets. It felt dreary.

It needed a lot of work, and it took us all of our six years there to get through all the projects we'd mapped out when we moved in. After a complete kitchen remodel, new hardwood flooring throughout, and some paint here and there, it was finally the home we'd envisioned the day we moved in. I had only recently fallen in love with it, and now it was time to go.

With the house officially on the market, there was no time to waste. I needed to turn my attention to packing.

I poured myself another cup of coffee and made my way through the house, room by room, mentally preparing myself for a task that I never expected to be facing. *How exactly was I supposed to whittle my possessions down to only what would fit in that van?*

I immediately felt overwhelmed again. There was still so much to do.

To make the moving process easier, we separated the garage into sections. On one side, I staged items I wanted to take with me. And on the other side, he staged his. Down the middle, we placed any items that still needed to be discussed. At the front of the garage, near the doorway, we stacked up the items to be donated, which made the loading process easier.

For the most part, it was a smooth process. I wanted very few things that he wanted, and vice versa. On his side, there were piles and stacks of outdoor camping equipment, fishing tackle, tools, and other gear. And on mine there was home décor, kitchen gadgets, books, and clothing.

Occasionally, we'd come to an item that we both wanted to keep, and when it was possible, we'd simply divide it up. Wine, wine glasses, bath towels, kitchen knives—all were fairly easy to divvy up. But when it came to other things, like the Instant Pot or camping gear, we solved it by purchasing a duplicate on Amazon.

Our relationship had become mostly transactional, and for that I was grateful. We'd managed to limit our interactions to discussions about what to sell, donate, or toss. Being emotionally detached made the uncoupling process quicker, easier, and much less painful.

My packing strategy was to start with the big things, like furniture, garden tools, and larger pieces of home décor. Then, I moved on to sentimental items, such as holiday decorations, gifts from family and friends, and mementos I'd picked up on various trips over the years. Next, I tackled more functional items, like small kitchen appliances, office supplies, and clothes. After that, I'd have to see how much room was left in the van.

It became apparent right away that I wouldn't be able to take much in the way of furniture. At most, I could probably only fit one or two large pieces. Knowing that I could replace the furniture later, I focused my attention on the smaller items—things that were functional, held sentimental value, or items that would be difficult to replace.

The next part was fun. Once again, I walked from room to room, this time cherry picking items that I loved. I felt like I was on a shopping spree, loading up my cart with beautiful things without giving a single thought to the price tag.

I had to be careful, though. With the house on the market, potential buyers would be visiting soon, and I didn't want to disrupt the carefully staged rooms too much. That was another reason the garage became the staging area.

On my side of the garage, there were several storage bins stacked up along the wall. Most of them hadn't been touched since the day we moved in, and I needed to clear out the space so I could visualize how much stuff I was actually planning to bring in the van. The clutter was making me crazy.

I set up my sorting area, which consisted of a stool and two large containers—one for trash and one for donating. Then I got to work.

I tossed out my high school yearbooks, which I'd only cracked open a handful of times in the 23 years since graduation. They were heavy, and I couldn't justify them taking up space.

I tossed out several boxes of mementos—old high school love letters, blue ribbons, certificates of achievement, and other trinkets that felt pointless to keep. I knew they would just end up in another garage or closet if I kept them.

Into the appropriate bins, I tossed childhood Christmas tree ornaments, photos, cassette tapes, electrical cords, gardening supplies, and books.

I was ready to start over.

Even so, seeing our possessions scattered all over the cold, cement floor saddened me. Objects that once held significance were piled up, waiting to either be poured into the landfill or sold to strangers.

As I sorted, laughed, and cried my way through all the memories of my life, I couldn't help but wonder why I'd carried all that ridiculous crap around with me for so many years. Nothing came to mind. It had done nothing more than fill space, and space was a luxury I no longer had.

I could have never predicted that less than four weeks after our conversation on the couch, our house would be under contract. After being on the market for just five days, it sold for over asking price. It was a huge relief, especially from a financial standpoint. In the back of my mind, I'd been worrying about the possibility that we'd somehow lose money on the house. At least we would both be able to leave with a little bit of money in our savings accounts to start over.

I was grateful that the proceeds from the sale of the house would at least give me a cushion. I didn't have a steady income yet from my business, and our divorce agreement hadn't included alimony. I knew that as long as I could get through the first few months, I could figure it out from there.

But with the house now sold, I faced another tight timeline. Rather than the customary 30-day closing timeline, the buyers wanted to take possession in just 24 days. That was just three weeks away. That's all the time I had to figure out what to keep and what to release.

And I still didn't have the van.

# Downsizing

Three days later—just nine days after I wrote a check for the down payment on the van—my phone rang while I was out running errands.

"It's here," Lance said.

I inhaled sharply and held my breath, barely able to process what he'd just said. I couldn't speak.

"I'll see you within the hour," I said.

When I hung up the phone, my body relaxed immediately. It was the most relaxed I'd felt in weeks. Finally, my exit plan was starting to come together. I closed my eyes, feeling a deep sense of gratitude. I'd trusted that everything would work out. And so far, it had.

Not having to waste my precious energy worrying about whether the van would arrive on time was a huge relief. I no longer had to fret over making back-up plans. Finally, I could shift my focus completely to pulling my life together. And I had three weeks to do it.

I put the car in drive and did my best to focus my attention on the road, while I managed the swirling emotions in my head. It was surreal. Everything was happening so quickly.

I made a quick stop at home to clear out the last of my personal items from the car and pick up the second set of keys for the trade-in. Then, I headed toward the dealership.

When I turned into the dealership parking lot, Lance was already standing outside, and by the time I opened my car door, he and another service member were standing next to me.

"If you want to give this gentleman your keys, he'll work on getting your trade-in processed while we get started on your paperwork," Lance said.

I handed over my keys and followed Lance to an office inside the dealership. A blonde woman greeted me from behind a desk and invited me to have a seat in front of her. On the desk, there was a huge pile of documents, and I wondered how long it would take to get through it all. After a few signatures, the transaction was complete. I was finally the proud owner of my very own Sprinter van. I was officially a #vangirl who was about to enter the world of #vanlife. And I'd also just purchased the most expensive vehicle I'd ever owned at $55,697.50.

Lance returned to the office dangling the van keys out in front of him.

"Are you ready to get your van?" he asked.

I smiled in response and followed him outside, where my van was parked in front of the dealership. It sparkled in what little sun had peeked out from behind the clouds. I couldn't wait to sit down in the driver's seat.

When he handed me the keys, it felt like he'd handed me a new life.

The step up to the driver's seat was a long one. From the ground up, it's a solid 18-½ inches. I grabbed ahold of the steering wheel and hoisted myself up into the driver's seat. The scent of the brand-new interior was magnificent. I ran my fingers across the textured leather on the steering wheel. It felt luxurious.

While I'd driven the other van that we owned together plenty of times, this felt different. This one belonged to *me*. Over the past few days, I'd spent hours combing through my possessions, carefully curating a small collection of things that I adored. Soon, I'd be loading that collection into the back of the van.

At some point, Lance climbed into the passenger seat next to me and started pulling out booklets from the glove box. I hadn't noticed. I was already envisioning myself driving through the California desert.

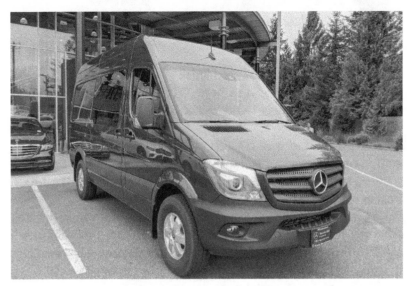

*Picking up the van at the dealership*

I slid the key into the ignition and turned it one click forward. When the glow plug light disappeared, I turned the key further until I heard the diesel engine hum to life. The dash lit up and the odometer showed 11 miles. Somehow that felt significant.

I'm fairly certain that Lance was trying to talk me through the features, but I was only pretending to listen. I was still processing the fact that I was sitting in what could very well be my new temporary home, and I was lost in a daydream.

I envisioned myself driving down the Oregon coast with the windows down. I imagined what it would be like to see the Grand Canyon. I thought about how I might feel staring up at the giant Sequoias. Besides, I'd already been through the same presentation when we bought the first van, and I didn't need the spiel.

I twisted myself around to look in the back. It looked smaller than I remembered, and my thoughts drifted back to my giant pile of possessions in the garage at home. I hoped it would all fit, but I feared that I was going to have to whittle down my collection even further.

I turned back around and looked out the giant front window, nodding to Lance as if I'd been listening carefully to his every word the whole time.

When it was clear that he'd finished going through his checklist, I extended my hand to him. "Thank you so much, Lance," I said. "You have no idea how much this is going to change my life."

We shook hands and he climbed down from the passenger seat, closing the door behind him.

I pressed on the brake, slid the gear into drive, and then eased the van out of its space. It had been quite a while since I'd driven the other van, and I'd forgotten how unwieldy it is. After maneuvering the monster through the dealership parking lot, I turned onto the main road and headed home. My head was buzzing as I drove in silence. I was trying to think about what to do first when I got back home.

With the van, at least I finally had a place to sleep, prepare meals, and store my possessions. With those essentials taken care of, it really didn't matter where I ended up after the house closed. I was one step closer to creating a new life for myself.

When I arrived home, I slowly inched the van up the gravel driveway, but hit the brake about halfway up. The van idled loudly as I tried to figure out how exactly to squeeze it into a spot. With the other van already parked in front of the two-car garage, it barely left any wiggle room for a second. It would be tight. Even if I did manage to get it parked, getting it out again could be just as tricky.

Shaped like a lowercase "t," the driveway was a challenge. The two shorter sides of the "t" were used primarily as turn-arounds. But even for smaller compact cars, it took some serious finessing to get it right. Any time we had guests over, it was comical to watch them leave. We'd wave from the front porch, giggling to ourselves as they made a series of 3-point turns.

I decided to aim for what looked like the easiest spot, hoping that one hard left turn would get me there. But since I was stopped on a slight incline, the wheels spun out briefly before the van finally started to move again.

When I thought I'd reached the right spot, I cranked the wheel hard to the left and prayed it would fit. I stuck my head out the window and looked behind me to make sure the back of the van wasn't too close to the giant western red cedar that was leaning out partially into the driveway. I barely missed it, and somehow managed to complete the turn. I judged it good enough, put the van in park, turned off the ignition, and set the emergency brake.

But before I could unfasten my seatbelt, tears were already rolling down my cheeks. I felt grateful. I was amazed by just how beautifully everything was coming together. All the big things on my list had been checked off. The house was sold, the divorce documents were filed, and I was finally sitting behind the wheel of what was, at least for a while, my new home.

Everything had been divinely orchestrated on my behalf.

When I'd finally composed myself, I stood up between the driver and passenger seats and looked into the back of the van. The high roof made the interior seem expansive, but I knew that once I started loading up my things, it wouldn't take long to fill the space. I walked into the back of the van and envisioned myself living there. In my mind I saw myself preparing meals in my kitchen, curling up into the soft blankets in my bed, and working with clients by phone at a small table. I had everything I needed.

I pulled out my phone and opened the Pinterest app, clicking on the board titled "Sprinter Love." As I scrolled through the images, I wondered if I could realistically pull off any of the buildout in the three weeks I had to work with.

I scanned through images of cozy beds with fluffy bedding, micro kitchens with sinks and fridges, and creative storage solutions that made use of every square inch of space possible.

But I'd have to consider that later. My brain felt like mush, and what I needed the most was rest. I closed the app, gathered my things, and walked toward the house to call it an early night.

The next morning, I pulled out my to-do list and scanned the remaining items still left undone. With just three weeks before closing, there was still a lot to do. Closets and bookshelves were still cram-packed full, four decades of knick-knacks were lurking in random drawers, corners, and bins throughout the house, and I hadn't even touched the outdoor shed yet.

In a way, three weeks felt like a gift. I'd worked myself up into believing that I'd have just a few days to frantically tie up all the loose ends of my life. Three weeks felt like an eternity.

As much as I wanted to start loading the van and playing with various configurations for my living space, I needed to carefully consider the order of operations. I didn't want to load up the van, only to find that it needed to be completely rearranged.

The garage was starting to look like it was inhabited by hoarders, and it was next to impossible to walk through it without knocking something over. The clutter was killing me, and I needed to get it organized.

To create more staging space, I figured it made sense to start by clearing out the donation bins that were already completely full. I loaded up the van with furniture, home décor, bags of clothes, and other odds and ends that we'd mutually agreed to donate, and then headed to the donation center.

When I returned home, I refocused my efforts on the inside of the house. I'd been dreading the task of sorting through my book collection, but I couldn't ignore it any longer. I had no idea how many books I owned in total, but I knew that I'd have to let go of most of them.

Why I'd felt it necessary to keep every single copy of every book I'd ever purchased, I had no idea, but I kicked myself for not transitioning to digital or audio formats earlier. As I stared at the five, 6-cubby Ikea bookshelves in my office, I knew it was going to be a serious downsizing job.

I decided to limit myself to just one box of books. That would have to do. With space being so limited in the van, there was simply no room to bring more. And if I ended up missing any of the books I parted with, I could just buy a digital copy later.

To get the sorting process started, I scanned each book title and pulled any that I felt a strong connection to. The first pass was easy. The Bible, *A Course in Miracles,* and *Loving What Is,* all made the cut, along with a few others.

Very quickly I realized that I needed to set some additional criteria to make the process of paring down the collection easier. First, any books that made it to the "keep" box would need to be ones that I'd reference again frequently. Second, keepers would also need to be books that weren't easily consumed in audio or digital formats, such as ones with worksheets or space for journaling. And third, any books that came along for the ride would have to be integral to my healing process on a personal level.

My plan was to take the books I wouldn't be keeping to Half-Price Books, a used bookstore that purchases used books. At least I'd be able to recoup some of the money that I'd invested over the years.

After a few more rounds of sorting, using the criteria I'd set, the box was full.

I loaded the remaining books into bins, boxes, and bags, and felt a twinge of sadness at the thought of parting with them. I still hadn't read some of them. At least fifteen books were "on deck," as I often called it. I had a habit of clicking the "buy now" button, even though I still had a stack of books in the queue ahead of them.

In the end, I have no idea how many trips I made to Half-Price Books, but I did at least manage to recover a couple hundred dollars.

In the brief moments when I wasn't sorting or packing, I thought about my future. I thought about what I wanted my life to look like, how I wanted to feel, and where I wanted to go on my trip. Those little moments of escape gave me the encouragement I needed to keep going.

With the van now in my possession, I could go anywhere in the U.S. easily. But that reality was also paralyzing. Most people dream about having the freedom to go anywhere, but having endless options felt terrifying. I had no clarity about where I wanted to end up, and I felt myself teetering toward the life of a wandering vagabond.

But regardless of where I ended up in the long run, I knew that I'd eventually need to make my way to the East Coast to visit my family at some point. They'd been understandably concerned about my well-being, and I knew that a visit would bring comfort to all of us. They needed to know that I was really okay, and I needed to be hugged by people who loved me. With that in mind, I added Ohio and Florida to my list of eventual destinations.

My mind then wandered to items on my bucket list—national parks, scenic highways, and other popular destinations that friends had raved about over the years. Crater Lake, Palm Springs, and Mesa Verde were a few of the places I'd added to my list in recent years.

In the back of my mind, I wondered if I might fall in love with a place somewhere along my trip. Maybe I'd arrive in a small town somewhere in the middle of the country and decide to stay.

Or maybe I'd fall in love with van life. I wondered if maybe I was destined to be on a perpetual rolling adventure, wandering aimlessly for the rest of my life. Other van enthusiasts had somehow figured out how to make their vans a permanent home.

In some ways, the idea of life on the road sounded easy. I mean, how hard could it be to drive around and find a parking spot? But the more practical parts of me knew that it was going to be trickier than that.

In just a few days I'd gotten really comfortable driving the van. Parking and making sharp turns were a cinch, and I'd mastered my mirrors like nobody's business. But I'm quite sure that I looked like a Muppet driving it. At just 5'1" my head barely reached the headrest.

On a daily basis, the song "No Roots" by Alice Merton blared from the radio. It had become my theme song. I felt like she'd written it for me. The peppy beat always seemed to lift my spirits, reminding me that maybe it wasn't so bad to be without roots. I knew that roots could be replanted. And I realized that maybe I could figure out a way to feel grounded without needing to stay in one place.

At least I hoped so.

Before I could begin loading the van, I still needed to complete a few projects. The van would have to be livable, so it was important that I planned the layout carefully, especially for the things I used on a daily basis. As I considered what I might need on the road, I made a list of a few essentials:

- A place to store food
- A place to store valuables
- A place to sleep
- An emergency toilet
- A way to cook
- A sink to wash dishes

Storage needs were solved quickly. I already had a small wooden hutch in the bathroom that would fit perfectly along one wall of the van. It was currently full of makeup and other bathroom supplies, but I'd have to go through it soon enough anyway. The hutch would need to be secured to the frame of the van, so it didn't tip over during travel. I had a few tie-down straps that I hoped would work.

One thing that concerned me was how to secure the few valuables and personal documents that I'd be bringing along. I didn't want my tax records, jewelry, or cash to be too easily accessible just in case I needed to have the van serviced at a dealership, or use valet parking somewhere along the way. While it wasn't fail-safe, I decided to buy a small lockable filing cabinet that could be hidden beneath the rest of my things.

Sleeping arrangements were also fairly easy. I already had a sleeping bag that could be placed right down the middle of the van at night. I'd have to be careful about how I loaded everything, but I was pretty sure it would work. For comfort, I planned to use an inflatable sleeping pad beneath my sleeping bag. The pad could be easily deflated during the day when I'd need the space to prepare meals. The only problem was the pad I already had was too small. I'd never replaced it because we'd recently purchased cots, making the pads unnecessary. But I needed something slightly bigger and more comfortable for a longer-term trip. I pulled out my phone and after a few clicks, a new one was on the way.

Next, I did a quick web search and found a simple portable toilet. It looked like a small gray bucket with a black lid, and it came with a few sealable "double doodie bags" that could be disposed of in a regular trash can, much like a baby diaper. I giggled as I added it to my Amazon cart. While totally unglamourous, it would serve its purpose in the event of an emergency. As an added backup, I'd also planned to join Planet Fitness, which would give me access to showers, along with another bathroom option, in a pinch.

Cooking was simple. Having nearly two decades of experience as a registered dietitian meant that I could throw a meal together with just about anything in a matter of minutes. And over the years, I'd cooked plenty of meals on our trusty, two-burner Coleman Triton stove. I also planned to pack some energy bars, along with some items that didn't require heating or cooking, like peanut butter.

The only thing left was a sink. While most campsites offered a source of potable drinking water, it wasn't always accessible. In most cases, a simple wash tub and some Dawn soap would probably be adequate. But with safety being a big concern for me, I didn't want to be wandering around a campsite after dark looking for fresh water to do dishes. And I also wasn't keen on the idea of doing dishes in the rain or when it was cold outside. Having a sink in the van would be so much more convenient, and it would make hand washing and brushing my teeth a whole lot easier, too.

I returned to my Pinterest board, scanning through images to see how others had handled their sink installation. It looked simple enough, so I decided to attempt building one myself. I'd settled on a gray water system, using a foot-pump and a small cabinet. My plan was to cut a hole in the top of the cabinet, drop in a small bar sink, and attach some beverage tubing to a couple of potable water containers that could be stored inside the cabinet. That way, the water would be well-secured for travel, and easily accessible when it was time to dump or refill the containers at the campground.

I knew I had to get started on the project soon, and I crossed my fingers that I'd be able to pull it off with my limited construction skills before the tools were packed up for good.

During one of my trips to Half-Price Books, I noticed a Pier

One next door, so I decided to stop in to see if they might have a cabinet that could work as the sink base. They were having a Memorial Day sale, which was a bonus.

I meandered through the store, examining the furniture displays closely, and mentally disregarding any that were too wide, too deep, or too long. What I needed was very specific.

And then I noticed one that looked promising. It was a simple, multi-colored wood hutch with a textured triangle inlay on the front. It was stunning and matched my vision perfectly for the future van buildout, whenever that might be. I located the tag, and saw that it was priced at $499.95. But on top of the cabinet was a giant red sign advertising a 20% off promotion. Score!

The only potential drawback I could see was that the two front doors fastened with a magnetic closure. I'd have to figure out a better way to secure it because magnets wouldn't be strong enough for travel. I dreaded the thought of water spilling out all over the floor of the van the moment I hit a pothole. Other than that, it looked like it just might work.

I found a store clerk and asked if he could help me load it up after I cashed out at the register. While he searched for a hand truck, I completed the purchase and headed back outside to the parking lot to bring the van around.

On the way home from Pier One, I decided to stop at Home Depot to see what they had in the way of sinks. I'd already ordered the foot-pump, drain, and water containers, which were at home in the garage waiting. All I needed to do to complete the project was pick up a sink and some beverage tubing. It seemed simple enough. Fortunately, there was one 6"-deep bar sink left in stock, so I wrangled it into my cart and continued on to find the beverage tubing. With both items that I needed now in my cart, I made my way to the checkout and headed home.

When I got home, my husband's van was parked in the driveway. He'd just returned home from a business trip, and I was grateful that he was willing to lend a hand with getting the cabinet out of the van. It was bulkier than I realized, and there was absolutely no way I could have moved it on my own.

We carefully lowered the cabinet down to the driveway, and I gathered the rest of my supplies. I wasn't even sure the sink was going to fit. I hadn't had a chance to measure anything yet. I'd relied solely on the eyeball method.

The first thing I checked was to see if the water containers would fit. I placed the two gray water jugs inside the cabinet and held my breath as I closed the doors. When I heard the metal closures click into place, I breathed a huge sigh of relief. They fit.

Next, I pulled the sink from the box and placed it upside down on top of the cabinet. It looked like it would fit. After carefully positioning the sink where I wanted it, I outlined my cut-line with a pencil.

Then it was time for the saw. Power tools weren't exactly my jam, mostly because I rarely had a chance to use them. For most of my life, a man has always stepped in and taken over projects before I could even get them started. It's like men can sense it the moment I pick up a power tool. But this project was finally mine.

I found the jigsaw in the garage, plugged it into the extension cord, and returned to the cabinet in the driveway. As I stood there with the saw in my hand, I realized that I first needed to drill some pilot holes in the top corners, since there was no opening to drop in the jig.

I dropped the saw to the driveway and I returned to the garage to search for a drill. After drilling four holes, I picked up the jigsaw again and began cutting along the pencil line. It took a lot longer than I expected to get through the wood, but finally the top piece broke loose and dropped into the base of the cabinet.

I lowered the sink into place and stepped back to take a look. It fit perfectly. With the sink securely in place, I attached the drain and then fed the plastic drain tube into the gray water container.

Next, I fastened one end of a piece of beverage tubing to the foot pump and the other to the cold water supply line of the sink. It wasn't as tight as I'd hoped, but it would have to do for now. With another piece of beverage tubing, I connected the other open end of the foot pump with the fresh water container. It looked right. But then again, I'd never assembled a sink before.

I'd already partially filled the fresh water container, so I could test the pump once I had everything attached. It was time to put it to the test. I turned the knob of the cold water tap to the on position and stepped down onto the round rubber pump cover. Nothing happened. When I looked down, I noticed a small puddle of water pooling inside the cabinet. There was a loose connection somewhere.

But I'd have to troubleshoot that later. I wasn't sure how long my husband would be home, and I wanted to get the cabinet back in the van while I had the chance. We carefully hoisted it back into the van and secured it with tie-down straps.

Hoping to get the project checked off my to-do list, I decided to head back to the hardware store to pick up the few remaining supplies I still needed—some plumber's tape, a few clamps to tighten the beverage tubing connections, and a connector for the cold water line.

After parking the van in the Home Depot parking lot, I grabbed a small piece of beverage tubing, just in case I'd need it for sizing, and walked toward the store entrance. When I stepped into the plumbing aisle, I immediately wanted to curl up into the fetal position. There were shelves and shelves of fittings—copper ones, steel ones, plastic ones. There were straight sections, T-shaped sections, L-shaped sections, and shapes that made absolutely no sense to me whatsoever.

Some fittings were bigger on one side and smaller on the other, and I realized quickly that I was going to need some help. I scanned the nearby aisles looking for someone wearing an orange apron, and finally flagged down a friendly-looking man.

"Hi Tony," I said, reading from his name badge. "I'm looking for a connector thingy," I said.

"Connector thingy?" he asked with a wide grin on his face.

"Yes," I said. And then we both burst out laughing.

"I have no idea what I'm doing, but I'm eventually going to have a working sink when this is all over with," I said.

After I explained to him what I was looking for, he motioned for me to follow him.

But without the cold water supply line to match up the fittings, it was next to impossible to determine which one I needed.

"I guess I'm going to have to buy all of these and bring back the ones that don't work," I said.

"Can you bring the piece in?" Tony asked.

"No, but it's right outside in my van if you want to come take a look," I said. I was pretty sure he'd say no. My guess was that it was frowned upon for store employees to hop into vans with strangers.

"Okay," he said.

"Well, okay then," I said.

When we reached the van in the parking lot, I slid open the side door.

"Wow, this is awesome!" he said. "How much was it?"

The van had been in my possession for less than a week, and he was the second stranger to ask me that question. I was somewhat surprised by just how bold some people were about personal questions like that.

"About $55,000," I said.

"Wow, I figured it would be more than that," he said.

I stepped up into the van and opened the sink base.

"You'll probably need to jump up here to see what I'm talking about," I said.

Tony joined me in the van and crouched down in front of the sink cabinet to take a closer look at the fittings. I hoped he couldn't hear me giggling behind him. I was trying to figure out how I'd just managed to talk a complete stranger into hopping into a random van in the parking lot.

"I think I know what you're going to need," he said. I hoped he was right.

We returned to the plumbing aisle and Tony promptly selected a handful of fittings.

"One of these will work," he said.

We headed back out to the van to test out a couple of the options.

"This one works!" he said excitedly.

We walked back into the store and when we reached the checkout line, Tony handed me the part. I thanked him for his time, and for going above and beyond to help me find what I needed, and then I took my place in line.

When I got home, I secured the new fitting with plumber's tape, attached the clamps, and held my breath as I stepped on the foot pump once again. After a few pumps, water began pouring out of the faucet and into the sink. I looked under the sink to check for leaks, but everything was dry.

It worked!

It felt damn good to know that I could do things on my own. Even if the sink wasn't perfect, it was done. And I'd done it with minimal help.

The van was still far from my Pinterest-inspired, bistro-on-wheels vision, but it was a start. Once I figured out where to settle down, I could search for a builder to complete the conversion. But at this stage, it just needed to be travel-worthy.

With most of the van essentials now in place, it was time to begin loading my stuff. I suspected it would take several trials before I found the right configuration that both maximized space and allowed me to access items I might need on the road.

# The Armoire

With the closing on the house just a week away, I'd successfully narrowed down my possessions to one pile in the garage. The pile looked much bigger than the space available in the van, though, and I feared I'd have to leave some of it behind.

I knew that once I loaded the van, there would be very little space for last-minute hauls to the donation center. The center aisle and the passenger seat area would be the only open spaces, so I needed to plan carefully.

Most of the bigger pieces of furniture had already been dealt with, but there was one item still left to consider: the armoire.

Made of a chocolatey dark wood, the armoire was another Pier One score from several years earlier when I lived in Austin. On the left side there were five vertical drawers with ring-shaped metal pulls, and on the right side a single door with a carved-out, triangular inlay.

Initially, I'd removed the armoire's hanging wardrobe rod and used it to store office supplies. But after I moved from Austin to Issaquah, it found a new home in the living room. For years, it lovingly held some of my most cherished possessions—my jadeite Fire King collection, a gift from my grandmother; my delicate Waterford Bassano china with its platinum-trimmed cream and pearl white pattern; and other family heirlooms that I only brought out only on special occasions.

Its stoicism was symbolic of the strength I so desperately needed, and I wasn't sure that I was ready to part with it.

I'd lie awake at night envisioning the possible Tetris moves I could use to somehow squeeze it into the van. I pictured it standing upright, lying on its side, facing down—but no matter which way I spun it, it wasn't going to fit. And even if it did, it would only mean that I'd have to give up something else in its place.

I'd already whittled my life down to the bare essentials, and I couldn't bear the thought of parting with anything else.

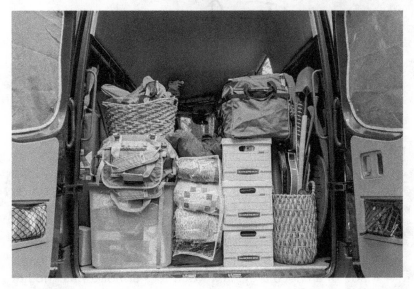

*Packing the van*

The idea of saying goodbye to the armoire was much more difficult than I expected. I wanted to force it to fit—because that's what we do when we aren't ready to let go. We force things to fit even when we know they don't. We file down their edges, saw off their legs, and disassemble them until what we loved most about them is lost. And sometimes we do the same thing in relationships. We try to change the people we love to make them fit our world, when really the most loving thing we can do is to let them go.

Yes, the armoire was beautiful, but like so many things in my life that had once seemed to fit perfectly, it was time to release it to someone else who wouldn't need to alter it. It was time to let it go.

Two days after I loaded the armoire into the van and dropped it off at the donation center, I woke up physically and emotionally exhausted. I was grateful that I'd had the sense to schedule a massage for early that Sunday morning. I needed it. My muscles ached, my skeleton hurt, and my brain was barely functional.

Monthly massages had become an essential part of my self-care practice. So much so, that I budgeted them as a separate line item under healthcare expenses. They really had become that important to my well-being.

My very first massage had been a gift from my husband on my thirtieth birthday. Afterward, I felt like a different person. I felt relaxed and grounded and balanced. But I also felt slightly disappointed. For at least ten years of my adult life, I'd carried an enormous amount of stress and anxiety that could have easily been dissolved in an hour on a massage table. I wished I'd known about them sooner.

When I arrived at the spa, the receptionist handed me a lavender-scented neck pillow, which she'd just pulled from the warmer. I placed it on my shoulders and made my way to the relaxation room, where I found a seat near a water feature that hung on the wall. The sound of the soft trickling water was so calming that I nearly nodded off twice before the therapist arrived to call me back to the room.

When I slid onto the warm massage table, my body melted into it. It had been exactly six weeks to the day since our conversation on the couch, and the 42 days in between had stirred up a whirlwind of change. It was hard to believe that in just five days, I'd be waking up at my home for the very last time. The stress and emotional intensity of it all had finally caught up with me. My body was in physical pain.

The therapist carefully worked out every tight spot in my shoulders and back, and by the time she made her way to my head, I felt a twinge of disappointment, knowing that the massage was nearing the end. Afterward, I felt better but I knew it was going to take some time before I felt good again.

I was finally feeling ready to close up this chapter of my life, and all the memories that came along with it.

# Empty

The day before closing, there were only a few things left to do: take one last trip to the donation center, do some last-minute cleaning, and do a final load of laundry.

I'd purposely planned a buffer day, so I wouldn't have to run around frantically trying to finish everything at the last minute. For me, feeling rushed ranks up there with feeling cold. I'll do just about anything to avoid either.

I rolled out of bed, slid on my slippers, and wrapped myself in my trusty, fuzzy robe before making my way down to the kitchen. I'd programmed the coffee machine the night before—something I had done for years. Being able to pour myself a fresh cup-o-joe as soon as I opened my eyes helped me ease into the morning.

After filling my mug, I walked toward the front of the house and looked out the window. It was still dark outside. I loved the quiet stillness of the early morning hours. When it wasn't raining, I'd often enjoy a cup of coffee or two on the swing.

I opened the front door and stepped out. The chilly air immediately stung my cheeks, but my robe kept me warm and cozy as I walked toward the wooden swing, which was nestled up against a few rhododendrons and azaleas. They'd be blooming soon, but I wouldn't be there to enjoy them.

And then I felt a wave of sadness wash over me when I realized that I also wouldn't be able to enjoy the hummingbird that often visited me in the spring and summer months. I'd usually hear the buzz of her wings long before I saw the flash of her color.

I was fairly certain she was a "she" because hummingbirds often return to the same location each year, and often on the same exact date. Around that same time a year earlier, I discovered a small nest in one of the rhododendrons out back. First, there were two tiny eggs, and then a few days later, two of the smallest chicks I'd ever seen appeared in their place.

But a late spring storm had blown through shortly after, and the chicks didn't make it. I was devastated. Less than a week before that, I'd lost all but one of my chickens to a hungry black bear. The past few years of my life had been full of losses, to say the least.

When my mug was empty, I returned to the house to map out the rest of my day. My husband planned to leave early that morning, and it would likely be the last time we would see each other.

It felt surreal to be saying goodbye. I felt grateful that we'd somehow managed to stay grounded while cohabitating over the past few weeks. His heavy travel schedule no doubt made it easier, and we had very limited interactions even when he was home.

And then it was time.

I stood in the empty room just inside the garage while he gathered the last of his things. I was still wearing my fuzzy robe and slippers, which shielded me from the cold tile floor below me.

We planned our uncoupling the way most people plan weddings—with careful attention to detail, yet with a strange sense of excitement about the future ahead. It was well-orchestrated. But even though I'd known the goodbye was coming, I felt completely unprepared.

And then it happened.

Our eyes met as he walked toward me. My heart stopped. I could feel the tears welling up and I wanted to throw up right there on the floor. As he got closer, he extended his arms and I immediately melted into them, just like I'd always done. It was a familiar place that I'd once felt safe. But it was different now.

We said what we needed to say, and then all at once he released me.

When the door closed behind him, I stood in the empty room—with nothing but my fuzzy robe left to console me.

I made my way to the living room couch, where we'd decided to end our marriage. Soon, I watched from the window as the first van we bought together, now towing a giant U-Haul behind it, inched slowly down the driveway.

Tears emptied onto my cheeks as the finality of everything hit me. Life would never be the same. In an instant, the taillights disappeared. And just like that, the man and the life that used to be mine disappeared right along with them.

When I'd composed myself, I found my journal and began releasing my emotions onto its pages.

*Thank you. I'm sorry. I love you.*

Those seven words summed up exactly how I felt about everything. I was truly grateful for the beautiful memories I'd be taking with me as I moved into the next chapter of my life. I was sorry for the role I'd played in the failure of our marriage. And even after everything we'd been through, I did still love the man who I'd soon be divorcing—just not the way I used to.

While things between us hadn't worked out quite the way I had hoped, it didn't mean that my life was over. As I closed the journal, it became clear to me that the next chapter of my life was just beginning.

With nothing left to do at home, I got dressed and headed into town to have breakfast at my favorite diner, Issaquah Café. The house felt cold and empty, and I suspected that moping around would only invite more bouts of crying. A change of scenery would do me some good, and with the kitchen completely packed up, cooking wasn't even possible.

When I arrived at the café, there was no need to look at the menu. I always ordered the same thing. The staff knew my order by heart: the California omelet with spicy jalapeno mango salsa and side of pumpkin pancakes.

After breakfast, I dropped off a few canned goods at the local food bank and ran a few more errands before returning home to finish up the last of the cleaning.

I'd decided to sleep in the van on my last night at home. Because I had to hand the keys over to the new owners by 9 a.m. the next day, it made sense to minimize my footprint inside the house. After the bedroom furniture sold, I'd been sleeping on a camp cot in the living room anyway, so I was basically indoor camping as it was. Plus, I was excited to get settled into my new tiny home on wheels. It was thrilling to be living so unconventionally.

At dusk, I did one last walk-through of the house. With the exception of the coffee pot, which I'd programmed to brew a final pot of coffee the next morning, everything was loaded into my new tiny home.

I stepped out onto the porch, locked the front door behind me, and made my way down the driveway toward the van.

After brushing my teeth for the very first time in the sink I'd just built, I laid out my sleeping bag on the floor and tucked myself inside it. It was quiet. And dark. And it was much colder than I imagined it would be. With no heat in the van, I zipped the sleeping bag up further around me and curled up on my side. As I drifted off to sleep, I imagined what my life would be like in the days and weeks to come.

In the morning, I awoke in complete darkness to the sound of birds chirping wildly outside the van. It was just after 4 a.m., about the same time I was used to getting up.

I unzipped my sleeping bag and braced myself for the chilly air. I grabbed my fuzzy robe, which was hanging from a nearby magnetic hook, and quickly wrapped myself inside it. After sliding my feet into my wool-lined slippers, I slid the van door open.

The cold air hit me instantly, rushing past me and filling the van. I could see my breath right away, and the little bit of heat that had accumulated inside the van overnight was gone now. I'd need to be careful in the future about opening the door too much. Using the passenger door might be a better option when it was cold. I'd have to file that away in my mental notes.

Over the years, I'd heard claims that Seattle winters are colder compared to other northern climates because of the rain. But having grown up in the Midwest, I was familiar with both kinds of cold. I didn't like either. Cold is cold.

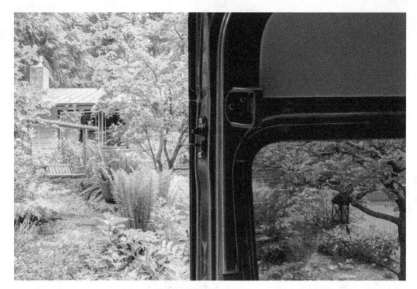

*A view of Stacy's swing from the van in the driveway*

I stepped down from the van into the driveway and walked toward the house, wondering briefly if any of my neighbors were up yet, and if they'd seen me get out of the van in my robe. If so, I was certain they must have been curious in recent weeks when they noticed two vans in the driveway instead of just one.

When I unlocked and opened the front door, the aroma of coffee greeted me. The house felt warm, a reminder of the comforts I'd soon be living without.

I walked into the kitchen and poured a cup of coffee into the mug I'd left next to the pot the night before. I swallowed hard, realizing this would be the last pot of coffee I'd ever brew there. In a couple more hours, the house would no longer belong to me.

I sat down on a stool next to the sliding glass doors in the kitchen, which opened to the back yard. The two white leather stools were among the few pieces of furniture the new buyers had arranged to keep.

From the sliding glass doors, I could see the tall western red cedars and Douglas firs. I remembered how neighbors had approached us soon after we'd moved in to ask if we'd be interested in cutting any of the trees down. We weren't. The trees were one of the reasons I fell in love with the property. In six short years, they had become my friends, inspiring me with their strength and groundedness. I wondered for a moment what they'd heard and seen while we lived there; they'd witnessed it all—every argument, every disappointment, every heartache.

I took another sip from my mug and wandered through the house room by room. Each held memories.

I remembered the day I got the key to the house six years ago. It was November, and I'd been living in a hotel while I waited for the house to close. My husband was still in Austin, handling the sale of our home there.

The move to the Seattle area had been prompted by a promotion I'd received at work. It was a whirlwind of change in a short period of time, not unlike the tornado I was moving through now.

The first night I spent at the new house, I'd laid out my sleeping bag in a corner of the master bedroom, where I slept for the first several weeks before our furniture was delivered from Austin. The thought occurred to me that perhaps I'd actually been camping out for the last several years; maybe I never really planted any roots at all.

I returned to the kitchen and poured myself another cup of coffee, and then made my way to my favorite spot in the front yard—the wooden swing that faced the driveway. It creaked as I sat down, a familiar sound that brought me comfort. At one point, we considered replacing it, but never got around to it.

My cheeks stung in the chilly morning air, but my robe and slippers kept the rest of me warm. Birds played out their usual morning symphony as I watched the steam from my mug swirl up in front of me. Red-headed pileated woodpeckers, chickadees, and robins were frequent visitors.

I took a deep breath. And then the tears came. It was hard to believe it was already closing day. Forty-seven days ago, I'd poured myself a cup of coffee like any other day.

And then my life changed in one conversation.

The chaos that surrounded the moving process was finally over, and for that I was grateful. But saying goodbye to the home

I'd grown to love was more difficult than I imagined. For weeks I'd been suppressing my emotions in an effort to stay focused on the to-do list.

Forever goodbyes are my least favorite. There's no good way to prepare for them. One minute, life exists in a series of safe, predictable routines. And the next, it's over.

As I sat crying quietly, I heard a familiar buzzing noise above my head. I recognized the sound instantly. When I looked up, there she was—my hummingbird friend—hovering right above me. From spring through summer, she'd visit the bright red flowers near the swing. Multiple times a day, she'd buzz around collecting nectar from the nearby fuchsia, Crocosmia, and other perennials that were planted throughout the landscape in the front yard.

She'd been through a lot, too. She'd experienced losses of her own. And yet, here she was again, still gliding through the air, collecting nectar, and moving on with her life.

I felt a knot in my stomach when I realized this would be the last time I'd ever see her. "Goodbye, my friend. Goodbye," I said out loud as more tears spilled down my cheeks. I was tired of saying goodbye.

When my mug was empty, I knew that it was time to go. But I didn't want to. I wanted to sit right there in the swing and preserve the beauty of the landscape, my home, my life.

I inhaled a chilly breath of air and stood up, the swing creaking beneath me. I took one last walk through the yard. I said goodbye to the first trillium of the season, with its tiny white bloom just barely opening. I said goodbye to the hellebores, with their blooms pointing downward toward the earth. I said goodbye to my favorite tree, a Kousa dogwood, whose prominent white and green flowers were just beginning their spectacular seasonal bloom. I said goodbye to my black raspberry canes that would just be coming into their first real fruit-bearing season. I said goodbye to the rhododendrons, with their endless bright red and pink buds. It was time to say goodbye to it all—including the future I'd once envisioned for myself there.

After a quick shower and one last walk-through of the house, I returned to the kitchen. I rinsed out my coffee mug in the sink and unplugged the coffee pot from the wall, carrying it with me as I walked out the front door.

I locked the door behind me and descended the stairs of the front porch for the last time, dropping the coffee pot in the garbage can in the driveway on my way to the van. I wasn't going to need it for a while, and there wasn't any space to spare in the van.

It was time to go.

I climbed into the driver's seat of the van, turned the ignition, and slowly eased it down the driveway for the last time. Stopping for a moment at the end of the driveway, I took one last look at the house from my rearview mirror, before mentally closing that chapter of my life forever.

As I turned out onto the main road, I remembered the first day that I drove through Issaquah with my realtor. I knew instantly that I wanted to live there. The quaint downtown shops, the tree-covered mountains in the distance—everything about it felt like home and I knew that I wanted to plant my roots there. But now I had no roots. I'd been uprooted.

I had no idea where I was going, but I hoped that someday I'd feel that I belonged somewhere again.

Right now, I was homeless.

# Saltwater

For my first night on the road, a friend that I'd met a few years earlier at one of my book club events was gracious enough to invite me over for dinner and to spend the night at her home. Closing day had been emotionally draining, and I was grateful for her friendship. Not having to be alone that first night helped make the transition easier. Having someone to talk to about all the swirling emotions I was experiencing was helpful. I was tired of crying and was grateful to have the distraction.

After dinner, we spent the evening chatting about where I might go on my trip, when I'd be returning to Seattle to finalize my divorce, and whether I might end up circling back around to the Pacific Northwest when my van adventure was over.

After leaving my friend's house the next morning, I grabbed some pumpkin pancakes at my favorite breakfast spot and began searching for a place to camp for the night. A small campground in Des Moines, WA called Saltwater State Park caught my eye. It was located along the Puget Sound between Seattle and Tacoma, and it had some amazing views of the water.

On the way, I stopped to pick up some block ice for my small Coleman cooler. I'd learned from earlier camping trips that block ice lasts longer and isn't as messy as regular bagged ice.

The van had officially become my home, but I couldn't venture far. I only had temporary tags from the dealership, and I had to wait for my permanent license plates to come in before I could leave for good.

In truth, I was grateful to have the extra time. I needed to get used to the idea of living in a van before I traveled too far away from my familiar surroundings. At least I had a few people in the area that I could call if I got into trouble. But the further away I ventured, the smaller my safety net would be. I planned to use the extra time to map out my trip and figure out where exactly I wanted to go.

It occurred to me that I might end up traveling for a few weeks, and then decide to loop right back around to Seattle. I was leaving it all open, mostly because I felt directionless.

When I arrived at the campground, the park ranger at the gate instructed me to drive through the campground and select any open site. Then, I'd need to return to the gate to complete the reservation card and submit payment.

Site #11 was open, so I quickly scribbled down the information on my reservation card and drove back to the front gate to officially reserve the spot. When I returned to the campsite, I wasn't quite sure what to do with myself. It was the first moment I'd really had to relax since the whirlwind began.

I felt hungry, so I pulled out my folding wooden table and chairs and set them up next to the van. There was a picnic table available, but the grass was tall and wet, and I didn't feel like lugging all my supplies across it if I didn't have to. Besides, I loved my little wooden table and chairs. It felt like home.

Once I had everything set up, I prepared a simple dinner of chicken noodle soup and a salad, along with some leftover crusty bread from lunch. It was chilly outside, but I felt warm and comfortable in my fleece.

I wanted to shower before bed, since I'd learned the very first night while camping in my driveway just how brutally cold the mornings were. I gathered up my supplies—a pair of flip flops, a change of clothes, a pack towel, and a bottle of Dr. Bronner's, which doubled as body wash and shampoo—and headed to the closest showering facility. When I walked in, I noticed that someone was already using the single outlet to charge a battery, which meant I wouldn't be able to plug in my blow dryer to dry my hair. Wet hair is a deal-breaker for me. It takes forever for my hair to dry on its own. If I go to bed with it wet, it will still be wet in the morning. And with temperatures dipping down into the 40s overnight, I knew I'd just lie there shivering all night. I'd have to settle for dry shampoo.

I stepped into the shower and locked the door behind me. But after I undressed, I discovered that special tokens were required for hot water. Not wanting to shower in cold water, I mumbled a few curse words under my breath and got dressed again to go in search of shower tokens.

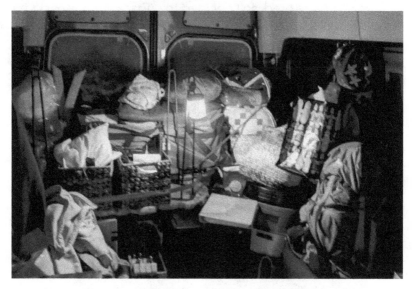

*The lantern-lit van at night*

Just outside the restrooms, I found the token dispenser. Fifty cents would give me three minutes of hot water—except I realized that I hadn't brought any money with me to the showers, which meant that I'd have to walk back to the van. Thankfully, the shower was still open when I returned with a handful of tokens.

By the time I got back to the van after my shower, it was almost dark. I locked the doors and grabbed the small solar-powered lantern that I stored on the dashboard during the day, where it could charge in the sun. It provided just enough light for reading.

After laying out my sleeping pad and arranging my sleeping bag on top, I poured myself a glass of wine and plopped down on my bed, resting my back on the sink cabinet.

In the back of the van, my possessions were stacked carefully and secured with an absurd number of bungee cords in varying sizes. All the fragile pieces of my life were secured by elastic. While it may have been unconventional, the van felt like home. Locked inside the large metal box, I felt safe. It wasn't the fancy layout that I'd envisioned on my Pinterest board, but it was mine.

I wasn't quite tired, so I decided to unpack my box of books. I couldn't remember what I saved and what I tossed. It felt like Christmas. Inside the box, I found eleven books:

- *Loving What Is* by Byron Katie
- *No Mud, No Lotus* by Thich Nhat Hanh
- *Animal Speak* by Ted Andrews
- *Nature and the Human Soul* by Bill Plotkin
- The Bible
- *A Course in Miracles* by Helen Schucman
- *Think and Grow Rich* by Napoleon Hill
- *The Tawny Scrawny Lion* by Kathryn Jackson
- *By the Waters of Babylon* by Stephen Vincent Benét
- *The Four Agreements* by Don Miguel Ruiz
- *Permaculture: A Designers' Manual* by Bill Mollison

I scanned each cover but none of the titles jumped out at me, so I returned the books to their box, and took another sip of my wine. My brain was at capacity and there was no room to absorb any new information. What I needed was to get some things out. I grabbed my journal and began filling several pages.

After spending several minutes releasing my thoughts onto the pages of my journal, I felt lighter, but I also felt sleepy. I could tell that temperatures outside were dropping because I could see my breath, so I decided to tuck myself in for the night. Since it was my first real night of camping alone, aside from the night that I camped in my own driveway, I wasn't sure what to expect.

While my new sleeping pad was more comfortable than the old one, it was still a bit narrower than I'd hoped. I had to position my arms and legs carefully, or they would slide off the edges and onto the cold floor beneath me. The only thing between my sleeping pad and the bare metal floor of the van was a thin rubber mat, which didn't offer much protection. On several occasions, I was jolted from my sleep after a wayward arm or leg would move the wrong way. To avoid this, I'd tuck my blankets up under my arms and do my best to be as still as a mummy.

I slept down the middle of the van like a sausage link until around 4:30 a.m., when the songbirds broke into their morning cacophony and made it impossible to sleep any longer. I felt more rested than I had the day before, but I already dreaded the idea of having to move to another campground. The amount of time and energy it took just to find a campsite, make reservations, drive to the site, check in, and get settled in, could easily take three hours.

So, over coffee I decided to simplify everything by staying another night. The van was easy to move, so it wouldn't be an issue to move to another site if someone else happened to have reserved my current one. Plus, staying put for another day would give me more time to get my bearings and come up with a plan.

I spent my day journaling, crying, and drinking tea, while simultaneously considering some possible travel destinations.

When the sun was out, I could at least keep the sliding door open and enjoy some fresh air. It wasn't quite like sitting in my little wooden swing at home, but it was close. With temperatures nearing the 60s, it was beautiful.

I decided to begin mapping out some ideas for the next place I'd like to settle down. I had blank slate to work with, and I came up with the following list of requirements:

- Warm + little-to-no snow
- Near a Planet Fitness, gym, or yoga studio
- 3- to 6-month lease available
- International airport within 1 hour
- Near a healthy grocery store or farmers' market
- Surface parking available for the van
- A Porch/balcony
- Green space for walking/hiking

It was a solid list. And when I couldn't think of anything more to add, I put down my pen and sat back to review the list. That pretty much summed up my requirements. At some point, I'd have to think about which cities and areas of the country fit that criteria.

By the end of the day I didn't feel much like cooking, so I found a nearby burger joint on the map and took a quick drive to pick up a to-go order. After dinner, I situated myself once again on my sleeping pad and tried to perfect my mummy technique.

The next morning, I crawled out from under my blankets and immediately put on my fuzzy robe. It was cold. Again. And I was thankful that I'd thought ahead and set up everything for my morning routine the night before. Before bed, I'd filled my teapot with water, added ground coffee to the French press, and staged everything on the sink counter near the door. That way, I'd have everything I needed when I opened the door and the blast of cold air hit me in the face. Getting a hot cup of coffee as quickly as possible was vital.

After putting on my slippers, I opened the sliding door and set up the camp stove. While the water was boiling, I had just enough time to put away my bedding and clear out some space for breakfast. After pressing and pouring myself a cup of coffee, I pulled a container of Ellenos Lemon Curd yogurt from the cooler and warmed myself with the liquid from my mug. The yogurt tasted like dessert, and the coffee felt like home.

Cleaning up after meals was my least favorite thing about van life, especially after breakfast. I loved my French press, but cleaning it was not even close to fun. Because I didn't want to risk clogging up my sink drain, I had to take a few extra steps than I would have had at home. First, I carefully scooped out the coffee grounds into a plastic bag with a paper towel. The first few times, this left me with coffee grounds all over my hands, and all over the van floor. After cleaning up my mess, I'd have to hand wash the carafe in the sink. And on days that I made an extra afternoon or evening pot of coffee, I had to go through the entire process again.

My mind drifted to the van build. I imagined the layout and décor—a beautiful, cozy cottage on wheels. I'd already spent months and months imagining a buildout for the other van, and now that I no longer had to compromise or gain anyone else's approval, everything was back on the table in terms of config-uration, so I needed to reconsider everything.

Knowing that I still had a few weeks before my license plates would arrive, I realized that I might have enough time to find a local builder to do at least part of the van conversion before I left on my trip. It wasn't optimal. Even if I was lucky enough to find someone, I'd have to find a storage unit for my things, as well as a temporary place to stay while the work was being completed.

To explore the option, I called two builders in the area and asked about their pricing and availability. That idea quickly fiz-zled. The prices were outrageously out of my budget, even for some of the most basic features I wanted, like insulation and a roof fan. And full buildouts teetered toward 100k. If the price wasn't shocking enough, both shops were scheduled out for months, one for almost a year, and they weren't accepting new projects.

I could see why so many people were attracted to camper-vans. I mean, who doesn't want to venture off into the woods periodically for a few days and leave the daily grind behind? More and more of my clients had started choosing vacation des-tinations that didn't have access to phones or the internet, simply so they wouldn't be bothered by frantic colleagues, demanding managers, or unreasonable clients.

Van camping offers benefits that, in my opinion, far outweigh RV camping or tent camping. For me, it's the sweet spot. Vans are easier to maneuver than RVs and take less time to set up than tents. And since it doubled as my daily driver, it was also cheaper than owning an RV.

Compared to tent camping, the van was much cleaner, more comfortable, and far safer. I liked being able to lock myself in the van at night. I felt less vulnerable. And if I ever encountered trouble, I could easily just hop in the driver's seat and drive away. That's not possible in most RVs, since they have hoses, wheel chocks, stabilizers, cords, slide outs, and other accessories that have to be taken care of before packing up and leaving.

After I concluded that even a partial van conversion wasn't going to be realistic before my trip, part of me was relieved. I wasn't exactly excited about having to coordinate another big transition so soon. I was tired of juggling all the pieces of my life. What I really needed was some rest, and I could make do with the temporary amenities I had in place. Plus, it occurred to me that I might even change my mind about which configuration I wanted after spending a few weeks on the road.

I still had no idea where I would end up. If I chose to settle down in a tropical climate, like Florida, I'd need to install a roof-top air conditioner. But if I ended up in a colder climate, I'd need a heater. My approach to the buildout would depend on a lot of factors that I simply couldn't predict yet. And there was no point in rushing it. One of the reasons I chose to buy my own van was to give myself time to decide what I really wanted without feeling rushed.

# Lake Easton

After spending two nights at Saltwater State Park I was ready to move on and explore some new places. I'd been curious about another campground further east near Cle Elum, a popular destination for campers. I booked a site online for one night and started my drive. I'd camped in remote locations before, but never alone. This would be a good way for me to ease into camping further away from the conveniences of the city. I'd be doing it soon enough, regardless of my readiness.

Lake Easton State Park sits at the base of the Cascade Mountains on more than 500 expansive acres. When I arrived, a ranger greeted me at the gate, and I entered the park to find my site for the evening. The campground was mostly empty. In some parts of the country, June marks the beginning of warmer weather, but not so much in the Pacific Northwest, especially at higher elevations. Overnight temperatures can easily dip into the 30s. And without insulation or heat in the van, I was essentially sleeping inside a folded-up piece of aluminum foil. It was cold. Really cold.

To avoid feeling frozen overnight, I began experimenting with a few different layering techniques. I'd start with a warm base layer of long underwear, wool socks, a beanie hat, and zip-up fleece. Then, I'd put on my robe, which was a bit bulkier than I liked, but it offered another layer of insulation. Plus, it had pockets to keep my hands warm. Next, I'd layer on a crocheted afghan that could be neatly tucked around the edges of my cocoon to keep the draft out. There was nothing worse than feeling a blast of cold air in the middle of the night. After that, I'd zip my sleeping bag around as much of the pile as possible and top it off with two layers of quilts on top. Then I'd pray that I wouldn't have to pee until morning.

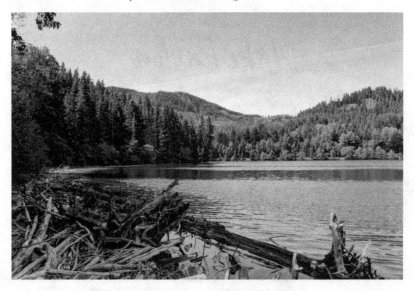

*Lake Easton State Park*

The past two nights had been so cold that I shivered myself to sleep, and I'd started to make a second pot of coffee in the afternoon just to take the chill off. My favorite coffee mug helped keep things light, though. Across the front were the words "classy, sassy, and a bit smart assy." I smiled every time I poured a cup. My mom always chose the best gifts.

At dusk, I locked myself in for the night and rummaged through my van wine cellar—a duffle bag collection of Cabernets and Semillons that my ex and I had divvied up before the move. I never imagined drinking them alone. Each one carried a memory of a special trip or experience, which almost always triggered a crying session.

One bottle of Semillon Blanc reminded me of a trip we took to Napa on our 7th wedding anniversary. I fell in love with it during a tasting at Stag's Leap Winery, so we ordered a case of it. Another bottle was a Jordan Cabernet Sauvignon, the same vintage as the year we were married. We'd plan to save it for our 10-year anniversary, but I no longer had a reason to save it. I popped the cork and poured myself a glass.

I smiled as I thought about the irony of drinking such an amazing bottle of wine while sitting on the floor of a van.

I slid out my box of books again, and pulled out *Loving What Is*. I needed a reminder that everything in my life was unfolding just as it was supposed to, that my suffering was optional, and that everything really was going to be okay.

I needed to remember Katie's simple wisdom, that everything that happened should have happened simply because it did.

The books that I'd carefully selected to be spared from the donation bin were books that offered me hope. Their words helped me reframe all the messy, difficult experiences I was still sifting through.

As I drifted off to sleep, I wondered once again how I'd ended up homeless and living in a van. A part of me wondered how I'd ended up so lucky. It really was an amazingly unusual adventure. While I certainly had to adjust everything about my day-to-day life, I was soaking in the peacefulness around me.

When I woke up the next morning, it was cold. Again. Still wrapped in my robe, I glanced in the mirror that was hanging by a hook above the sink. I looked like I'd just crawled out of a dumpster. My hair was staticky and I had a streak of mascara under each of my eyes. Evidently, I'd forgotten to wash my face before my evening cry session. I was still forcing myself to get dressed and put on makeup every morning. I felt better when I did.

Getting into a new daily routine was difficult. Even though I only had a couple of days of camping under my belt, I'd figured out that no two days were ever the same. For most of my life, I'd thrived on routine, but nothing about my life was routine now. Every campsite presented a new set of options and amenities, and every day brought a new set of weather conditions. I had to adapt to whatever came my way.

Before I found myself living in a van, my morning self-care practice had always included journaling. It gave me a chance to reflect on the wins and challenges from the previous day, and to get clear about what I wanted to accomplish in the day ahead.

But I noticed that there were fewer and fewer wins logged in my journal. Instead, I was investing a lot of energy trying to reconcile what exactly had happened to my life and what led to the unraveling of our marriage.

I wanted to blame my husband for my unhappiness. I wanted to blame him for the end of our marriage. And I'd devoted years of my life to punishing him for his indiscretions. I punished him subtly with my words, ensuring that he hadn't forgotten about our secret. But I also punished him with my constant state of sadness. I rarely felt joyful, and part of me wondered if I'd purposely withheld it from myself as a form of punishment to him. After all, victimhood had become part of my identity.

After breakfast, I couldn't wait to get back on the road, mostly so I could crank up the heat. But also because a friend of mine who lived in the Tacoma area had invited me to spend the night at her home. She had a small camper of her own, and we'd planned to go camping together the following night. I was grateful to have a warm place to shower and a place to sleep for the night that didn't involve shivering myself to sleep, even if it was only for one night.

On the way back toward Seattle, I stopped to use the bathroom at a rest stop near Lake Easton. A patch of sunshine caught my eye in the distance, and I made my way over to a small bench near the water's edge. I sat down and closed my eyes as the warm sun blanketed me. And I envisioned a future that didn't involve me having to constantly fight to stay warm.

Back on the road, I thought about my trip. I'd pretty much settled on Florida as my final destination. Since I already had family there, I knew that if I didn't find a place somewhere along the way, I could at least stay with them temporarily. Plus, Florida was warm. And that was one of the few criteria that I'd come up with as I considered the next place to call home.

My plan was to use Florida as my end point and leave everything else open. I didn't know if I'd be on the road for a few weeks or a few months, or whether I'd love it so much that I'd never want to plant any roots. That thought frightened me a little. I never saw myself as a full-time van dweller. It was more of a means to an end, even if I didn't know what that end was yet.

With my final destination decided, I thought about which cities I might want to visit along the way that might be potential permanent locations.

I thought about the Carolinas. I have family in the area, and I've enjoyed past visits to the mountainous areas, like Asheville, Hendersonville, and Lake Lure. I also really enjoyed vacationing at Myrtle Beach and the Isle of Palm. The beach sounded nice after so many cold nights. I'd never been to Raleigh, but for some reason I was drawn to it, so I added it to the list of places to visit at some point along the trip.

# Debt Free

When we decided to end our marriage, one of the things I was most grateful for was that we were completely debt free. That made the uncoupling process much easier.

We'd eliminated our debt back in 2008, just three months after completing Dave Ramsey's Financial Peace program, and we'd managed to stay that way since. I remembered how liberating it felt when I paid off that last credit card. I no longer had to worry about minimum payments, credit card interest rates, or whether I could qualify for a loan. Being out from under the rock of financial debt was such a gift.

Being financially free simplified everything. Because carrying a balance almost always means paying more than the actual value of something—in the form of interest and other hidden convenience fees—I'd learned that being debt free prevented me from overpaying for things.

And it also saved time. I hadn't realized how much time I spent each month writing checks and balancing accounts, not to mention the time I spent fretting over whether or not there would be enough money in the bank to cover everything.

But the purchase of the van had put me back into debt. And I instantly felt the weight of it after I'd signed the paperwork back at the dealership. With my share of the proceeds from the sale of the house, my plan was to pay off the loan as soon as the funds were available in my account. I'd have just enough money to pay off the van and still have a small cushion to carry me through for a short time while I traveled and searched for a place to settle down permanently.

In the interim, I rented a small mailbox at a local store just before the house sold. That way, I'd have a place to receive mail during the transition. And if I wanted to have my mail forwarded to some other location, all I had to do was call.

On a daily basis, I checked my bank account balance to see if the funds had posted yet, and visited the mailbox to see if the first bill for the van had arrived. As soon as my account balance showed sufficient funds, I planned to be debt free again.

A few days later, on the very same day, both my bank funds and the first van invoice arrived. I immediately called the loan company to verify the payoff amount. I had hoped I could make the payment electronically, but I learned they only accepted cashier's checks by mail.

I'd never mailed a check of that size before, so the idea of sending it through the mail made me feel a bit uneasy. Anything can happen to mail in transit. Because my father is a retired US Postal Service letter carrier, I'm probably a bit more trusting of the USPS than most people. But still, a lot was riding on that check arriving.

I secured a cashier's check from my bank, placed it in an envelope addressed to the loan company, and drove straight to the post office. I decided to opt for tracking, so I'd at least know when it arrived, but I wasn't sure if I'd be able to get insurance on the check.

I stepped up to the window and the clerk behind the desk greeted me warmly as I placed the envelope and tracking slip on the counter in front of her.

"Would you like insurance?" she asked, as she typed the information printed on the front of the envelope into her computer.

"Well, it's a check," I said. "So, I'm not sure what my options are." I wasn't sure if they could even insure a check, or if they could, whether there were limits on the amount.

"How much is the check for?" she asked, still staring at her computer screen.

"Just a little over $46,000," I said.

She turned and looked up at me from her computer, her eyes widened. "The most we can insure is up to $5,000, but..." she leaned over toward me from the counter and whispered, "Obviously I can't guarantee anything, but we rarely have problems with checks arriving."

I completed the transaction, left the check with the clerk, and prayed that it would arrive without incident. I had enough to worry about, and decided to release the outcome to the universe once again.

*Whatever will be, will be. Que sera sera.*

In the days that followed, I called the loan company repeatedly to see if the check had arrived. And a few days later, I breathed a sigh of relief when my account status was marked "paid in full."

Debt-mother-fucking-free.

*Check.*

# Tinkham

Feeling relieved about paying off the van, I was ready to celebrate. I'd made plans to spend the evening with my friend Amanda, who had also been our realtor. She greeted me with a smile when I arrived at her home, and my body felt warm the moment I stepped inside.

I felt grateful that she'd been available to help with the sale of our home. She already knew my backstory, and that made everything easier. I didn't have to explain my unique challenges or special requests, and she was incredibly compassionate every step of the way.

I'd only been on the road camping for three nights, yet I hadn't realized how much I missed the creature comforts of home. Just sitting in a real chair felt luxurious.

Our plan was to spend one night at her house, so I could unwind after being on the road for a few days. I needed to do some laundry and take a real shower that didn't require flip flops. Then, the next night we'd find a large enough campsite that would accommodate both her pull-behind camper and my van.

We spent that evening talking about everything from meditation to manifesting the life experiences we desired deeply. It took some time, but I'd built some wonderful friendships over the past three years. Having a strong support network had been more important that I realized.

We arrived at Tinkham Campground, which was just a little over 30 miles from what used to be my home, just before dusk the next day. Since it was a Wednesday, it was mostly empty, and we pretty much had our choice of sites. We chose one that looked large enough and positioned our vehicles so that our entryway doors opened to each other. I waited in the van while Amanda set up her camper for the night. There was nothing for me to set up.

Afterward, we decided to take a short stroll before dark. Amanda's cute little dog, Bella, needed a walk, and we wanted to enjoy as much of the scenic landscape as possible before the last bit of daylight fell below the tree line. The campground was nestled alongside the South Fork of the Snoqualmie River, which offered amazing views of the surrounding mountains.

It was the kind of view you often find in travel magazines, or hanging from the walls of art galleries. But being there in person was an entirely different experience. The view was one thing, but breathing in the damp, earthy ground beneath me, and the aromatic evergreens above me only intensified the experience. It was spiritual. I knew that if I did decide to leave Washington State permanently, I'd miss seeing the lush green forests and rivers.

Back at the campsite, we could still hear the faint sound of rushing water. I thought of Zoey, and how she was supposed to be with me on this trip. She would have loved exploring the area with me. And she probably would have helped keep me warm in the cold van. On a daily basis, I thought of her, and of how different my life was now, compared to even just a few weeks earlier.

As soon as we set up our chairs outside, it started raining, so we opted to move inside her camper, which was already warm from her propane heater. I was secretly jealous that she had access to a source of heat with just the switch of a button.

The more days I spent on the road fighting to stay warm, the more I realized that I'd spent most of my days feeling cold since I'd moved here from Austin. I took hot showers daily. I stayed wrapped up in my fuzzy robe most of the time. And I wore slippers around the house for at least ten months out of the year. Maybe it really was time to consider settling down somewhere warmer.

We spent the evening playing cards, drinking wine, and listening to 80's music until we laughed so hard that I nearly peed my pants. We clinked our glasses to the fact that I was debt free. Freedom in general had become a new theme for me.

Eventually, our eyes grew heavy, and when we couldn't keep them open any longer, I said goodnight and headed back to my van.

I dreaded it. The cold air that surely awaited me was a far cry from Amanda's warm and cozy camper. But it was my home now. And I was going to have to get used to it. When I closed the door behind me in the van, I could see my breath. I changed clothes as quickly as I could, and began my usual, albeit laborious, layering process.

The next morning, we returned to Amanda's house in Tacoma. Since I hadn't made any reservations yet for camping that night, she invited me to stay another few nights. I was grateful to have the extra time to plan my next mini camping trip.

I scoured the internet searching for campgrounds I might like to explore next. I wished I could venture further than just a few hours. My license plates were the only things standing between me and the open road, and I was growing eager to get moving—away from the memories of a city that I once fell so in love with, and away from the life I'd created there. But until the plates arrived, I'd have to find some places to camp locally.

I thought about boondocking for a while. Sometimes referred to as stealth camping, boondocking is where you find a low-profile spot to park overnight for free. It's not ideal for rule followers like me since laws vary throughout the country. Some cities are more tolerant, while others have strict laws prohibiting overnight public parking. Boondockers are left with the constant worry of the dreaded "2 a.m. knock," where an annoyed local resident or police officer will insist that they move on. That way of life never sounded appealing to me. I didn't need any more stress than I already had, and I don't like the idea of wondering if I'm breaking a law. And I definitely don't like to be disturbed from my sleep.

I much preferred the safety and amenities that campgrounds had to offer. It's just that my options for local campgrounds were limited. The ones closest to the city were extremely pricey, some over $100 per night. And at that rate, I could have just as easily sprung for a warm hotel. Most of the more reasonably priced campgrounds were several miles outside the city—further than I wanted to travel.

I also considered some other options, like asking a friend if they'd be okay with me parking overnight in their driveway. I was afraid they'd invite me in, though, and I didn't want to impose any more than I had to.

And then I remembered a woman that I'd recently met named Mitzi who owned a retreat center in the area. It was right down the road from my old house, and I wondered if she'd be okay with me spending a night or two in her parking lot. I sent her a message and waited for a response. Soon, I received her reply. She invited me over to chat.

When I arrived at her retreat center later that day, we ended up spending the evening sitting outside near the small pond that was situated on the property. During that conversation, I decided that July 4th—Independence Day—would be the day I would make my departure from Seattle. If my license plates arrived by then, that is. It seemed like the perfect day to officially reclaim my independence. And it was only two weeks away.

Rather than sleeping in my van in the parking lot, I was invited to stay the night at Mitzi's center, where she had three guest bedrooms available. I was grateful to once again have a heated place to stay for the night.

The next morning, I awoke with a strong sense of optimism. I felt grounded. I felt calm. And I was relieved to have finally settled on a departure date. As long as my license plates arrived before then, I'd be good to go. Everything felt like it was coming together, and I finally had something to look forward to again.

Later, Mitzi arrived back at the center and we had coffee together. During our chat, I decided to hold my official going-away party at her retreat center on July 1st, just a few days before my official departure.

# Beef Jerky

In the days that followed, I roamed from place to place—back to Amanda's house, then to a campground, then back to the retreat center. I spent a lot of time daydreaming about what I wanted my new life to be like, now that I had a completely blank slate to start over with.

During the day, I'd consider possible destinations to add to my itinerary, while I cried and ate beef jerky in the van. If that's what freedom looks like, then hella I was livin' the dream. Grieving...with beef jerky.

Crying was a daily ritual that offered at least some release for the intense energy that still came in surges. Aside from journaling, it was one of the most effective outlets for my emotions. The slow release of the tension that I'd been carrying for months felt amazing. Little by little I was relaxing into my new life. And little by little I was feeling more and more like myself again.

Being homeless was strange. Conveniences that I had taken for granted for so long now felt like luxuries: hot showers, wifi, push-button coffee. Even in just the first few days, the experience was humbling. I'd only been on the road for a little over a week, but that was long enough to appreciate that the life of a nomad isn't for the faint of heart.

I felt more gratitude for life's simplest comforts. I felt more compassion for those who hadn't chosen homelessness and didn't have the option of sleeping in a van. I'd become more keenly aware of everything around me, on high alert since I'd left the safety of home.

My intuition became my guide. Every choice I made was, at least on some level, made with my safety in mind. What time of day I showered, how I parked the van facing outward at campgrounds in case I ever had to leave in a hurry—every decision I made had been through a "what if" or "just in case" scenario first. I was still living in survival mode.

The van felt smaller and more cluttered than the cute images I'd pinned to my Pinterest boards. I guessed that most people who showcased their vans in photos weren't storing the entirety of their possessions in their van.

Several times, I attempted to rearrange the contents, but I couldn't find a way to make everything look cute while also having access to everything I needed. Everything had a spot, but there were no spots left.

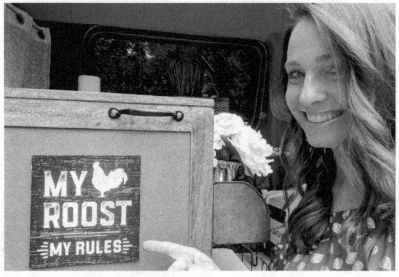

My roost

The only real décor in the van was a framed piece of art that I found at Hobby Lobby a few days after picking up the van. On the front was a picture of a rooster, along with the words

My Roost, My Rules. I knew the instant I saw it that it was destined to be mine.

I had to constantly remind myself that my living conditions were only temporary, that I'd eventually have a place to store my things, and that someday the van would align with the vision I held in my head. But right now, it looked more like I was having a yard sale.

While I longed for the cute bistro on wheels I'd been dreaming about, I also felt grateful. I was grateful that I wasn't completely without shelter. I was grateful that I had a safe place to store my things. And I was grateful that I hadn't decided to waste thousands of dollars moving hundreds of dollars of my possessions across the country. I had options, and that's what I was most grateful for.

# Penrose

Even so, I was getting tired of camping at the same camp-grounds. So, when a friend recommended Penrose Point State Park, I booked a reservation online for two nights.

When I arrived at the campground, I once again noticed that very few sites were occupied. I was still slightly ahead of season, which generally kicked off around Independence Day. Weekend dates were starting to fill up, but the weekdays were still pretty wide open.

After I parked the van, I unpacked my table and chairs and placed them in a patch of sunlight near the back of the van. Having grown used to the elusive Pacific Northwest summers, I'd learned to find random sun patches whenever I could. They were rare, and they faded quickly. But I loved feeling the warmth of the sun on my skin, and soaked it up every chance I got.

While rearranging a few items in the van, I noticed a few beams of sunlight were streaming through a light catcher hanging from the rearview mirror. The pendant was made from a series of clear and purple beads, a feather-shaped shell at the center, and a large Swarovski crystal that hung from the base. The sunlight sparkled across the walls of the van, turning the pendant into a tiny disco ball that made me smile.

I'd purchased the light catcher several years ago from a shamanic healer in Seattle. She made each one by hand, explaining that she allowed each pendant to name itself once it was complete. This one was named Faith. And faith was one of the few things I had left to cling to.

When the treetops near the campsite began fading out the sun, I decided to search for an open space where I could warm myself. I found a nearby trail and made my way over to the picnic area near the water's edge of Mayo Cove. I didn't very often wander far from my campsite for safety reasons. Traveling alone made me feel vulnerable. I didn't have anyone to lean on for support if I needed help. But because it was mid-day, and because I'd seen a few families at the campground when I arrived, I felt comfortable taking a walk.

When I emerged from the trail, I spotted an empty picnic table in the distance that was in full sun. I headed that way, and as soon as I sat down, I heard them—screaming bald eagles circling above me. I smiled in recognition. They seemed to find me no matter where I went, reminding me of my freedom, strength, and resiliency.

But still, I couldn't escape the sadness. It lingered. It continued to paralyze me, holding me hostage. One moment, I'd be smiling, and the next tears would be flowing down my cheeks without warning. I wasn't sure if the sadness was still due to mourning the loss of my marriage, or if it was related to something else. After all, I'd lost more than just a marriage; I'd lost a life.

The end of this relationship felt different compared to the end of my first marriage. Starting over in my twenties was inconvenient, sure. But at least I still had plenty of runway in terms of earning years. It eased my mind to know that I still had some time to make up for the financial losses that came with the end of that partnership. But starting over in my forties felt different. I recognized that my runway was shorter, and the idea of starting over again felt more daunting than I expected.

An older couple at a nearby picnic table caught my attention. They were eating lunch together overlooking the water and speaking a language that I didn't recognize. On top of the picnic table sat a small green and white metal cooler, and in front of each of them was a sandwich and a can of soda. I wondered what they'd been through in all their years together. Had they ever disappointed one another? Was divorce ever an option that they'd considered? Had they ever been to therapy? How had they managed to work through all the chaos of married life? And, perhaps more importantly, were they truly happy still?

My thoughts drifted back to family stories I'd heard as a child. I'd been told that my great-grandmother once said, "If I'd have known how to drive a car, I'd have left him years ago." I was certain she'd said playfully, but part of me wondered if there was some truth behind her words. Maybe past generations had been more invested in the idea of marriage out of necessity. Farming was hard work, and it would have been impossible to do alone. Maybe younger generations like mine just had more viable alternatives.

Crows began to circle overhead, and I noticed one was carrying a hot dog. It looked like a giant cigar hanging out of the side of its beak, which made me giggle. More crows descended on a nearby picnic table that was unattended—the source of the hot dogs. One by one, crow after crow descended on the picnic table and flew off with its own cigar. I admired their resourcefulness. They were masters of opportunity. Before the picnickers even realized what was happening, the hot dogs were gone.

I walked the short trail back to the van to prepare for my evening routine. Some of my most memorable camp meals so far included a medley of fresh fruit, cheeses, vegetables, and crusty bread with olive oil and balsamic vinegar. It reminded me of a trip my husband and I took six years earlier. Back in 2012, just before moving to Issaquah, we spent three weeks exploring five European countries in a rented campervan. Most nights, we'd gather up a few ingredients and some wine from local markets, and then piece together a random meal that reflected the flavors of the region we were visiting.

Looking back, I realized that trip was probably a big reason I was drawn to van life. It had most certainly prepared me for the spontaneity of life on the road, and likely gave me the confidence to know that I could do it.

In the past two weeks of my introduction to solo van camping, simplicity became my aim. The more I simplified, the easier life felt. And more ease was what I so desperately wanted.

# More Saltwater

Since I still hadn't received my plates, I decided to return to Saltwater State Park. It was close to the main highway. It was clean, campsites were plentiful, and at just $25/night, the price was hard to beat. But little by little, my days were consumed by small tasks that left very little left for planning or actual work on my business. Even my daily routines, from showering to washing dishes, took longer than they had at home.

A friend who lived near the campground invited me to her home to have dinner with her family. It was nice to have some social interaction. I hadn't realized how disconnected I felt, even after just a few days of wandering. After dinner, Stephanie gave me a tour of her almost-finished she shed, which her husband was still putting some finishing touches on. It was beautiful. And it reminded me of the van, which I was eager to get back to before dark. Being away from it for any length of time made me feel anxious. The thought of it being broken into had become an increasing worry. If it were ever stolen, I'd lose everything.

The next morning, while journaling with the van door open, I heard the familiar sound of a hummingbird. Looking up from my journal, I saw it hovering above some flowers at the edge of the campsite. It reminded me of my swing, of my home, and of the life I'd left behind. As it fluttered from flower to flower, my mind wandered back to my hummingbird friend in Issaquah. I missed her.

Van life wasn't everything I hoped it would be. There were moments when I questioned my decision. I wasn't sure I'd be able to pull off a cross-country trip on my own. I worried constantly about everything from theft, to running into a mechanical problem in the middle of nowhere, to being harassed by a stranger.

Everything—and I do mean everything—took longer. Filling up fresh water containers, emptying gray water containers, showering, preparing meals, doing dishes, making coffee, doing laundry, spreading out and folding up the bedding, rearranging the contents of the van. Everything took more time than it had at home, and the days and nights seemed to melt away faster on the road.

At night as I drifted off to sleep, I'd imagine a future that included a plush queen-size mattress with ultra-soft sheets. It was all I could think about while lying on the cold floor of the van. But this experience did at least give me the opportunity to reassess all the things that mattered most to me. It showed me which things I missed, and which things I didn't.

When I originally envisioned what life would be like on the road, I thought I'd have a lot more time to write. I figured I'd be able to crank out blogs on the daily, and perhaps even start writing a book about the experience. But I was lucky to have a few hours here and there at best.

Some days, when I left the door open, strangers would approach me to ask questions about the van. It was usually the traditional RV owners that had the most questions. Many were considering making the switch to a van because of storage fees and maintenance costs associated with larger campers. But those seemingly casual chats would often turn into hour-long conversations. Bit by bit, the minutes of the day ticked away, and I had little to show for it.

My self-care practice looked different, too. While my morning routine mostly remained the same, consisting of meditation, journaling, reading, and completing the Rate Your 8 assessment in my *Lifestyle Design Planner*, there were a few other areas that I had to rethink.

For physical activity I had to get creative, taking short walks during the day when I felt safe to do so. I also had a yoga mat that I could unroll in the space where I laid out my sleeping bag. It was tight quarters, and I couldn't do any radical poses, but at least I could stretch. I also had a pair of ten-pound dumbbells tucked behind my driver's seat. So, even if it was raining, I could do stretching and strength training exercises.

I was also grateful that the few coaching clients I had during that time were so understanding. They ended up getting a front seat view of my trip as I shared videos and photos regularly. Self-care wasn't just something I talked about and wrote about, it was something that I lived.

But with very little time to spare, I realized I didn't really have sufficient time to add more clients. I'd have to wait until I found a place to settle down before I could really focus on expanding my business. For the time being, I had to focus on the clients I already had and plan out some future programs.

# Bill

Most campgrounds, especially ones in state and national forests, had little to no internet access, so I had to plan my work-related tasks carefully. Just before closing on the house, I'd expanded my Verizon plan to allow for more data while traveling. I wasn't sure how much more I'd need, but I didn't want to be stuck without it in case of an emergency.

There were some benefits to having less connectivity, though. Being without wifi kept me from getting sucked into the social media vortex, which allowed me to stay focused on my highest priorities: thinking about where I wanted to eventually settle down and figuring out where to go with my business.

On the days that I didn't have to travel to another campsite, I'd often find a warm coffee shop where I could access wifi and recharge my devices. When I was lucky enough to find a table next to an outlet, I'd plug in my phone, laptop, and portable power bank. While I was able to charge my phone when the van was running, whenever I spent several days at the same campsite, I had to rely on the power bank, which is why I wanted to keep it charged as much as possible. It was important to have a backup source of power.

No matter what time of day I arrived, coffee shops always seemed to be full of people. And people can be distracting. One day at a Starbucks, I overheard an especially entertaining conversation:

"How long have you been married, Bill?" asked the man in the ball cap.

"Sixty-two years," Bill replied.

"To the same woman?!" the man in the hat asked as he chuckled and glanced over at the third man in the group.

"Yeah, and nobody should ever be married that long," Bill added, laughing.

I laughed, too—so loud, in fact, that I had to quickly look down at my phone and pretend not to be paying attention to their conversation.

For a few more minutes, I sat listening to the three men talk about chores, projects, errands, and trips they were planning— and that's when Bill noticed my Sprinter van parked outside.

"See that van there?" he asked the others. "You put in a couple of beds, a sink, a refrigerator..."

*Yes, Bill, do go on.*

"That's all you need," he said emphatically.

*So right you are, Bill. So right you are.*

"Why don't you buy one, Bill?" asked the man in the hat, clearly the instigator in the group.

"Trouble is," Bill explained, "she'd want two of 'em."

More hysterical laughter broke out.

*You have no idea how right you are, Bill.*

Later that night I rigged up my laptop to watch my favorite movie, Romancing the Stone. It just doesn't get any better than stale popcorn and nostalgic movies in a van. The van felt cozy, a little bit like home.

It was the first time I'd ever watched a movie while camping. Aside from a random YouTube video here and there, I hadn't watched any TV. Quite honestly, I didn't miss having a TV blaring in my ear all the time. The silence was calming. I'd instead gotten used to skimming news headlines on my phone whenever I wanted to catch up on what was happening in the world. For that matter, I could have probably just eavesdropped at a coffee shop to stay up to date.

I didn't mind being alone. As an only child, I was used to inventing things to do by myself. For me, alone was never synonymous with lonely. But I was still trying to find the right balance between connection and solitude. I knew that I needed to maintain connections with friends and family, while also giving myself enough space to sort everything out.

The following day, I headed back to my friend Amanda's house, which had become my second home whenever I wasn't camping. She'd planned a small gathering of friends as a sort of pre-going-away party for me. I wasn't sure when I'd see any of them again after I left on the trip, and I hadn't really had much time to plan get-togethers.

Spending the evening with friends was incredibly soul filling. We drank a few glasses of wine and laughed about some of the fond memories we'd made in the short amount of time we'd known one another. By the time the evening ended, I was tired, and my cheeks hurt from all the laughter. I needed that.

I needed to be surrounded by positive, encouraging people who believed in me. Friends give us the courage and strength to do things we might not do otherwise.

# Willie

I spent the next 8 nights at my friend's retreat center. Since I'd be leaving for my trip in a little over a week, and had already planned to have my going-away party there, she invited me to stay in the interim. It was therapeutic on a number of levels.

It was comforting to know that I'd be staying in one place for a while. I'd been homeless for just two short weeks, but it seemed like months. It had taken a lot more out of me than I realized. I was exhausted, and I needed to get my bearings before the real trip began. Sleeping in a real bed had evidently improved the quality of my sleep because I felt more rested than I had in days.

Being on the road made me feel vulnerable. I hadn't realized that I'd been carrying so much tension. But being on constant alert and hyper aware of my surroundings took a lot of energy.

The back porch of the retreat center overlooked a small pond, where I'd spend time journaling and planning my trip. On several occasions, I heard the familiar hum of a tiny hummingbird. I wondered if it was the same one that used to visit me regularly near my swing, which was just a little over a mile up the hill.

Knowing that I was so close to my old home was comforting in some ways. Everything felt familiar. But it was also heartbreaking. I missed my home, and being so close to it made me miss it even more.

Each day, I'd pull out my road atlas and add some new potential destinations to my Seattle-to-Florida itinerary. Aside from stops to see family, every stop on my wish list that I felt excited about seemed to be west of Texas.

The next morning, I scheduled a facial at a local spa. I'd intentionally left the afternoon open for self-care. I'd gotten so much better at managing my energy levels since my focus on self-care first began. I was better at recognizing when I needed to rest, when I needed connection, and when I needed solitude.

Before my facial appointment, I stopped in at a nearby Planet Fitness to sign up for a Black Card membership, which would allow me access to every Planet Fitness throughout the country. Other van dwellers had highly recommended the card, saying that it was an essential resource. Not only was it a great way to stay physically active on the road, but it also offered a place to use the shower if you were unable to access one otherwise.

After my facial, I stopped to have lunch at a little café in Gilman Village called The Boarding House. I loved the quaint dining room with its antique furniture and décor. It reminded me of my great-grandmother's house. After a turkey sandwich and a bowl of dill potato soup, I headed back to the retreat center.

But on the way, I remembered that it had been months since I'd visited Willie.

A year earlier in the spring, a black bear had climbed the fence to our back yard and destroyed the chicken coop, leaving only one hen behind. Willie was a beautiful, Red-Laced Wyandotte with beige and light brown feathers. She was the sole survivor. Somehow, she'd managed to escape the bear.

I suspected it was because she'd spent her entire life fighting to survive. We'd named her Willie because when she was just a tiny chick, the other chicks constantly pecked at her. So much so, that we thought she'd be blind in one eye—hence the nickname One-Eyed-Willie. Chickens don't do well alone; they need to be around other chickens. Fortunately, I found a home for her. Fox Hollow Farm, a nearby rescue farm and event center agreed to take her in.

I pulled into the mulch-covered parking lot at Fox Hollow Farm, but after I put the van in park, I couldn't get out. I felt sick.

I wondered if Willie would still be there, and I wasn't sure how I'd react if she wasn't. She'd been through so much. So had I.

It was just one of the many painful memories I'd collected in the six short years I'd lived in Issaquah. Loss after loss. Disappointment after disappointment. It left me feeling numb.

I stepped out of the van and walked toward the entrance of the farm. As I walked, I searched for Willie, crouching down to look beneath low-growing bushes and shrubs, and scouring the other groups of chickens that were gathered throughout the property. But didn't see her. I asked a couple of the staff members if she was still there, doing my best to describe her coloring. They hadn't recalled seeing her.

And that was that. Willie was gone, just like everything else in my life that once brought me joy. Gone.

Feeling the heaviness of yet another loss, I walked slowly back toward the van, allowing tears to stream freely. I was half surprised I had any tears left. I said a silent prayer, hoping Willie had somehow escaped again and had found a safe place to live in the wild.

Then I pulled back onto the main road and continued on to the retreat center.

# The Plates

The next day, I received the call I'd been waiting for. My plates had finally arrived, and were available for me to pick up at the dealership. I immediately jumped in the van, eager to get that important item crossed off my to-do list.

Finally, I had the green light to go. With just a week left before my official departure date, I could focus on securing a few last-minute supplies and mentally preparing myself for a cross-country trip.

It occurred to me that now that the plates had arrived, I was free to leave for my trip earlier if I wanted to. I considered canceling my going-away party, which was still four days away, and moving up my itinerary.

But I realized there was no need to rush myself. There were still some things I wanted to do. I wanted to go to the farmers' market one last time. I wanted to taste pumpkin pancakes one last time. And I wanted to see my friends again, since I didn't know when I might see them again.

I recommitted to my Independence Day departure and returned to the retreat center, where I began creating a music playlist that was a good fit for a cross-country journey, complete with songs about ended relationships and new beginnings. "All Out of Love" by Air Supply, Fleetwood Mac's "Gypsy," Mazzy Star's "Fade into You," and "Elastic Heart" by Sia were among the first few songs to be added to the playlist.

I felt caught somewhere between wishing my marriage hadn't ended and fighting to recover my own sovereign strength and independence. But each day, I grieved a little less. And after each bout of crying I felt a little stronger.

# Going Away

On my last Saturday morning in Issaquah, I decided to take a final stroll through the farmers' market. The rows and rows of beautiful flowers never ceased to amaze me—and they were extremely inexpensive. Most of the bouquets were around $5, and you could easily get a giant bunch of peonies for under $20.

The produce was impressive, too. But with limited space in the van, I couldn't buy much. I stopped and purchased a basket of figs and a small container of honeycomb, which I planned to pair with some blue cheese and crackers later that evening. Then, I continued making my way through the rest of the market while I silently whispered my final goodbyes.

As the day progressed, my body was signaling to me that it had reached its limit. The anxiety about my upcoming trip, the pressure of putting together the final details of my going-away party, which was set for the following day, and the lingering sadness that I still felt about everything that was changing in my life—it had all finally caught up with me.

I had a sore throat, my back ached, and my head felt dizzy.

Several weeks prior, I'd made plans to attend an event with a friend in downtown Seattle later that night, but I knew I was going to have to cancel. All I wanted to do was lie down, and I feared that if I pushed myself further, I might become too ill to travel.

I felt awful, and I must have looked the part because when I returned to the retreat center, Mitzi noticed the ridiculous state

I was in, and immediately called her personal massage therapist, Janene, to arrange for her to come give me a private massage at the center that evening.

Just before Janene arrived, I'd been instructed to take a bath, so I could warm my body and ease into a calmer state. When I emerged from the bathroom, she was setting up her massage table in the foyer just outside the door. It was getting dark outside and the room was mostly dark.

She greeted me with a warm smile and instructed me to have a seat on a chair that was next to the massage table where she had prepared a foot bath.

I asked her if it would be okay for me to write her a check, so I could get the payment taken care of beforehand, but she simply said, "It's been taken care of."

I didn't know what to say.

"I'd really like to pay you for this," I said. "I believe in the flow of giving and receiving."

"Maybe this is an opportunity for you to receive," she said. "You know, sometimes giving and receiving don't happen simultaneously."

Tears welled up in my eyes. She was right. I didn't know how to receive. It made me feel uncomfortable, and there were many times over the course of my life that I'd even questioned my ability to receive anything, including love.

She held out a container of essential oils and instructed me to select one. I chose lavender.

As she gently massaged my feet, she asked how I was feeling, where I was experiencing pain, and if I had any medical issues that she needed to know about. Tears began flowing, which surprised me. I rarely cried in front of other people, especially strangers. But for whatever reason, I felt comfortable sharing openly with her. I told her about my recent life transition, about my plans to travel across the country in the van, and about how terrified I was about the uncertain future still ahead of me.

After the foot bath, she directed me to the massage table, where a heated mat was laid out on top. It immediately warmed my body as I eased myself onto it.

And then for the next two hours, Janene magically unraveled the tension that had been slowly building up in my body for weeks, if not months. It was the deepest state of relaxation I'd ever felt, and I was so grateful that she and Mitzi had gifted me with such an amazing experience.

When the massage was over, I was half asleep on the table. When I felt alert enough, I rolled off the table and eased myself into bed, which was just a few steps from the massage table.

The next morning, I still felt relaxed when I woke up. My body no longer ached. My throat was no longer sore. And I was grateful, because my going-away gathering was scheduled for 4 p.m. that day, and I wanted to be fully present, so I could spend some quality time with friends.

After coffee, I spent the morning with my head in my planner completing a mid-year review. It's an exercise that I do every year, somewhere around the first of July. It's a chance for me to press the pause button and reflect on the first half of the year, so I can course correct and adjust the second half. And the first half of my year had been a cluster fuck and a half.

Back in January, my goals for the year had included "adventures in the campervan" and "converting the van," but I never imagined I'd be doing those things alone.

It's funny how quickly our lives can change. We live with the illusion that we know how the future will unfold, forgetting that we are only at the helm. Winds can change. Storms can pop up at any time. And we have to figure out how to make it through whatever comes our way.

The previous three weeks I'd spent waiting on my license plates to come in felt like a gift. It had given me a chance to test out van life without having to venture far from my familiar surroundings. It also gave me a chance to see if I had the chops to handle the weirdness of van life. And it was, indeed, weird.

When friends began arriving at the retreat center for my going-away gathering, it buoyed my spirits. I opened up the van in the parking lot and gave mini tours to those who were curious. I answered questions about the stops I planned to make. And I eased the minds of friends who admitted they were worried about me. Clearly, very few of their other friends had ever lived in vans—more evidence of the weirdness that was now my life.

When the sun finally sank below the horizon, all the guests had gone. Mitzi and I were the only ones left. After putting away the leftover food and tidying up the center, we sat down to share a glass of wine and say our goodbyes.

It would be my last night staying at the retreat center. I'd booked a hotel for the night before my trip. I wanted to make everything as easy as possible for my first day of travel.

On July 3rd, the day before my Independence Day maiden voyage, I'd purposely cleared my calendar. I wanted to give myself plenty of time to tie up loose ends and finish up last-minute errands.

I checked my mailbox one last time, fueled up the van, picked up some ice and a few last-minute items at the grocery store, and then headed over to Lake Sammamish State Park. It was a place that I'd visited frequently when I needed some nature therapy. Located on the south end of Lake Sammamish, the park was almost always packed with people, especially on sunny summer days. And in Seattle, most residents agree that the 4th of July marks the beginning of the short summer season.

When I arrived at the park, there were kids playing on the playground, kayakers and stand-up paddle boarders on the lake, boats lined up at the boat launch, and people enjoying the sunshine everywhere.

The park was also where I saw my very first bald eagle shortly after moving to Issaquah. My husband and I had recently bought a drift boat and were enjoying an afternoon fishing on the lake when a large shadow cast over us. Out of the corner of my eye, I saw something hit the water, and then a bald eagle emerged carrying a fish.

Each time I'd visited, I almost always saw at least one bald eagle. Just like my hummingbird friend, I was hoping to have a chance to say goodbye to my eagle friends as well. I got my wish.

It wasn't long before I saw the familiar flash of black and white above me. Not one, but four bald eagles were circling over the lake. It was fledgling season, which made it more likely that I'd see even more eagles as I moved closer to the Olympic Peninsula the next day.

I looked at my watch and noticed that it was after four, so I made my way back to the van and headed toward the Silver Cloud Hotel in Bellevue, where I'd made reservations to stay overnight. I wanted to have a chance to gather my thoughts and get some rest. I had no idea what might lie ahead of me.

Leaving on Independence Day felt extremely symbolic. It marked a new chapter for me.

For the first night of my trip, I'd made reservations at a campground in Poulsbo, WA. Since it was a holiday weekend, I expected most campgrounds to be full, and I didn't want any surprises. Knowing where I'd be staying ahead of time took the edge off my anxiety. I no longer had friends to lean on. I was officially on my own.

For the second night, I booked a campsite at a state park in Ocean City, WA. But everything after that was completely open. I had no timeline and no concrete plans other than the end destination of my mother's house in Florida.

My loose plans involved deciding over coffee each morning where I'd go next, and trusting that my permanent destination would reveal itself somewhere along the way. I'd go wherever I was led, stop whenever something tickled my fancy, and find a place to camp whenever I didn't feel like driving anymore.

It seemed like a simple enough plan. And after the past few tumultuous weeks, I wanted my life to feel as simple as possible. I was slowly beginning to realize that life really was easy. I was the one who had been making everything so complicated.

I pulled out my planner to double check that everything had been checked off my list. In the morning, I'd be leaving on an open-ended Independence Day adventure.

Somehow, I'd managed to survive the past eleven weeks of chaos. My life had been turned upside down, yet I'd managed to hold myself together through it all.

As I sank into the cold hotel sheets, thoughts swirled in my head. I wondered where I'd end up going, what I'd experience on the road, and if I'd end up changing my mind halfway through the trip and turning back toward Seattle.

But for now, I needed to get some sleep.

# PART II:
## Design

# Independence Day

When my alarm went off at 5 a.m. the next morning, I eased myself out of the hotel bed and made my way over to the coffee pot. It was strange to have push-button coffee again. I'd gotten so used to using my French press, and I'd grown to love the rich, aromatic coffee it made. I'd even gotten used to the cleanup process that at one time made me mumble curse words under my breath. But the button was still a lot easier.

After a couple cups of coffee and a quick shower, I gathered the last of my things and did one last walk-through of the hotel room before I completed the checkout process on my phone and walked down to the van.

I felt queasy. But it was an exciting kind of queasy. Not the throw-up-on-the-floor kind of queasy. This time I was the one doing the leaving.

While I still carried some fear about what the road ahead might hold, I no longer felt like I was in survival mode. I had everything I needed to start living again.

I was debt free. I owned a van that was filled with things that brought me joy. I had a AAA membership in case anything happened on the road and I needed help. I had a solid self-care practice that I could lean into when life felt unbalanced. I had a powerful network of friends that I could call on if I needed to feel connected. I had a business that was making money. And I had some savings that I could tap into if necessary while I got back on my feet, wherever and whenever I decided to do that.

I reminded myself that I had resources, and it boosted my confidence enough to realize that I was ready to go. It was time to start redesigning my life.

The highway was mostly empty when I turned onto I-90 and headed west. It was a Wednesday, but since it was a holiday, morning traffic was much lighter than usual. The hum of the highway felt oddly satisfying. It was a sound I'd grown to love over the seven weeks that I'd owned the van.

The van may not have had a foundation beneath it, but it was my home nonetheless. I started to wonder if I'd ever need roots again at all.

As I drove toward the ferry, it occurred to me that it had been almost eleven weeks since the conversation on the couch. I'd spent eleven weeks trying to figure out how to live on my own again.

And all of it had led me to this very moment—the moment in time when I was officially leaving my old life behind and starting a new one—on Independence Day, no less.

When I arrived at the ferry entrance, I stopped at the toll booth to purchase a one-way ticket to Bainbridge Island, a place I'd been to many times over the past few years. It was a favorite weekend destination. Between the quaint boutique shops and locally sourced restaurant menus, it was a fun way to kill a few hours on a random afternoon, especially if the weather was nice. But in my six years there, I'd never made it any further west than Bainbridge Island.

Since I wasn't sure when I'd be near the Olympic Peninsula again, it seemed like a good idea to begin my trip in the upper left-hand corner of the contiguous U.S. and work my way down to the lower right-hand corner in Florida.

With my ticket in hand, I took my place in the queue for the 10:40 a.m. ferry. Several lanes of cars, trucks, and cargo vans were lined up waiting for the official wave from a crew member to begin the boarding process. Some people waited contently in their cars, flipping through newspapers, or scrolling on their phones, and others emerged from their vehicles, gathering outside with other passengers to pass the time with conversation.

I sat quietly, watching everything that was happening around me. Traveling alone had made me more aware of my surroundings.

When the brake lights in front of me disappeared, I put the van in drive and followed the cars in front of me onto the ferry. After parking the van, I followed the other passengers up the stairs to the deck. I wanted to take some pictures to remember the moment that I officially left my life in Seattle behind.

The ferry was full of cheerful, patriotic families who oohed and aahed over the Puget Sound landscapes. I couldn't blame them. Summertime in Seattle truly is magical. The skyline is basically made up of three layers—tall evergreen trees, high-rise structures, and blue skies—all emerging from a foundation of water.

I gripped the railing of the ferry tightly as it broke free from the slip. The cold air pierced my cheeks as we slowly increased speed.

As we drifted away from Seattle, I hurriedly snapped pictures of the Emerald City, doing my best to preserve in my mind the memories I'd collected over the past six years. Some were heartwarming; some were heartbreaking. I could feel tears welling up in my eyes, but the wind dried them before they ran down my cheeks. I was grateful for that. It gave me a moment to collect myself.

I watched as the Seattle skyline slowly faded into the distance while the snow-capped mountains to the west grew larger. Two chapters of my life collided—my past and my future—just like the fresh water and salt water colliding in the cold, brackish water circulating beneath me.

And just like that, my old life became a memory.

The ferry engine rumbled beneath me as if trying to administer CPR to my lifeless body. I felt calm, withdrawn even. I'd been waiting for this transitional moment for weeks, and I was surprised that I wasn't a little more excited. Maybe it was because I'd suppressed the grieving process for so long just to make it through those early weeks. I'd only allowed myself an occasional cry session here and there when I was alone, and I knew there was more yet to come. I wanted to give myself permission to experience my emotions fully, but I needed the time and space to do that.

In some ways, I wasn't even sure what I was supposed to be grieving. The loss of my marriage? The loss of my life? The loss of my dog, Zoey? The fact that I'd given away almost all of my possessions? The loss of my hen, Willie? My donated book collection?

The losses felt overwhelming and I didn't know where to begin. But I knew I'd eventually have to get through each of them, one by one.

As the ferry approached Bainbridge Island, I made my way back down to the parking platform. The van was still warm from the heater that I'd had on full crank less than an hour earlier, and I relished that I was able to set the thermostat to any temperature I liked. The van, as small as it was, offered me a strange sense of comfort. It felt like a sacred space.

When the ferry finally docked, I started the engine and followed the cars in front of me down the ramp. The island was just as I'd remembered it. As I drove past some of my favorite places, I thought about stopping, but quickly remembered that I didn't need anything. And I certainly didn't have the space to bring anything more with me.

I passed Churchmouse Yarns & Teas, a shop that carries a wide variety of luxurious yarns and specialty teas. It was a place that I loved to visit. Something about the way I felt when I walked through the door always made me feel at home. In the front of the store, there was a large table where locals gathered to work on projects, and I suspected it's also where secrets were shared. I'd only just begun to build a community of my own in Seattle, and now I was leaving.

Coffee sounded good, so I made a stop at Sluys' Bakery in Poulsbo. A friend had recommended it after I mentioned that I loved an occasional sweet treat with my coffee in the morning. I found a parking spot near the marina boat launch and walked a few blocks to the store front. The sun felt good on my face and it also felt good to stretch my legs, but the air was still cold.

I was relieved when I finally opened the bakery door, where the sweet aroma of baked goods greeted me like an old friend.

I settled on a maple bar and a plain cup of coffee. After squaring up with the cashier, I ventured back outside to an empty bench in the sun.

All along the street, American flags were prominently displayed in celebration of Independence Day. It felt odd to spend such a festive day alone.

Each time the door of the bakery opened, the sweet aroma of yeast and sugar made its way over to me, as if trying to lure me back inside for another treat. I finished the last bite of my maple bar, tossed the empty bag into a nearby trash bin on the sidewalk, and headed down to the park at the edge of the Marina. A few people were already gathered near the water's edge to watch boats and seaplanes drifting in and out of the marina. My coffee cup doubled as a hand warmer as I made my way back to the warmth of the van.

# Eagle Tree

RV parks are generally a bit pricier than campgrounds at state and national parks because they have more amenities, like full water and electric hookups. While I didn't really need any fancy amenities, aside from a clean restroom and shower, a recent storm on the north end of the Olympic Peninsula—often referred to as simply the O.P.—had forced several state parks in the area to close. That meant there were fewer choices for primitive campers like me. And with the holiday weekend being such a popular family vacation option, I felt lucky just to have a place to park for the night.

By the time I arrived at Eagle Tree RV Park and found my site, it was already time to settle in for the night. Having camped enough times to learn the hard way, I found that setting up my sleeping gear was much easier by daylight than by lantern or flashlight.

Once everything was organized for the night, I made a quick dinner and filled a crystal wine goblet with some wine from my duffle bag. Then, I pulled out my journal. I was surprised, and perhaps even slightly annoyed that I was still journaling about my sadness. It had been almost three months since we'd decided to divorce, and I felt slightly disappointed in myself that I hadn't been able to shake the sadness. At least the pages of my journal offered me an anchor, showing me where I was in the grieving process. It gave me comfort to know that I was at least allowing myself the space to experience what I needed to.

Soon, my eyes got heavy and I tucked myself into the blankets on the floor. As I drifted off to sleep, I heard the sound of fireworks in the distance. I knew it was going to be a long night. I relished my quiet time, and it was anything but quiet.

# The Olympic Peninsula

The next morning, I awoke to the faint sound of fireworks still going strong in the distance. During the night I'd tossed and turned, occasionally getting jolted awake by the sound of booming fireworks.

Seeing my breath in the van no longer seemed odd. I shivered as I peeled back the layers of my blankets, but I knew that it wouldn't take long to feel warm again once I was wrapped in my fuzzy robe and prepared a cup of coffee. While the water for my coffee was boiling, I did a quick meditation and then once again pulled out my journal.

My morning routine had become the foundation of my self-care practice. It helped me stay grounded and kept me focused on my priorities rather than sitting around complaining about everything I didn't like about my life. My practice was my lifeline, a road map that showed me where to invest my time and energy.

For breakfast, I prepared scrambled eggs on the camp stove, and then rummaged through the van to see what else I might want to have with them. I settled on two mini mixed-berry scones and some fresh figs that I'd picked up at PCC, one of my favorite local organic markets.

Excited to spend some time exploring the Olympic Peninsula before moving on to my next campsite, I cleaned up the dishes, took a quick shower, and made sure everything in the van was secure for travel. More than once, I'd forgotten to fasten a drawer or secure the sink basin, and I had to pull off to the side of the road to clean up the mess. That was a lesson I learned early and quickly.

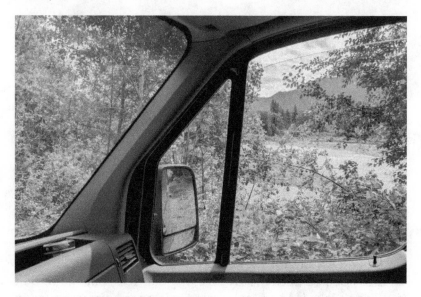

*The Hoh Rainforest on the Olympic Peninsula*

I wanted to at least drive through part of the Hoh Rainforest before I headed further south. One of the best purchases I'd made after buying the van was an annual national parks pass. For just $80, the pass would get me into any of the national park in the U.S., and it would eventually save me over $100 in the first couple of weeks of travel alone.

When I arrived at the entrance to the park, I flashed my pass to the ranger and rolled right on through. Easy peasy.

The Hoh Rainforest is remote. And rainy. And cold, barely reaching highs in the mid-70s at the height of the summer. But it's also one of the most lush, green landscapes I've ever seen, even compared to the island of Kauai or the beautiful Emerald City I'd just left behind.

Mosses of varying shades of green hung tightly to every-thing—trees, branches, rocks. I rolled the windows down and took a deep breath of the chilled, dewy air. With the exception of an occasional passing car and the sound of the van's tires thrumming against the pavement, the forest was quiet.

It felt like such a gift to be able to spend time there, in the stillness of nature. It was peaceful, the exact opposite of what I'd been experiencing over the past few weeks.

I wished I could stay longer, but I wanted to make a stop at Ruby Beach, a popular destination that friends had recommended, on the way to the next campground, which was still a little over two hours away.

# Ruby Beach

I meandered through the rainforest as long as I could to ensure that I could still make it to the campground before dark, and then I headed south toward Ruby Beach.

When I pulled into the parking lot, I managed to score a parking spot near a cliff overlooking the beach. I slid open the van door as my jaw simultaneously slid open.

Below me, the Pacific Ocean's waves lapped against the shoreline, where a few people were walking. They looked like tiny ants from above. Rock formations of all sizes and shapes jutted up from the ocean floor in every direction. Even from the cliff I was staring down from, they looked enormous. The gray sky and light layer of fog made the beach feel even more mysterious.

I followed some other beachgoers down a path that I guessed led to the beach, but I stopped when I reached an overlook near the midpoint of the trail. At every turn, there seemed to be a view that begged me to snap a photo.

At the bottom of the trail were hundreds, if not thousands, of pieces of driftwood. The massive tree trunks, which had been pushed up onto shore by the fierce ocean waves, looked as if someone had emptied a can of Pick-Up Sticks on the beach. I crawled over them carefully and made my way down to the shoreline. It dawned on me that if Zoey had still been with me, it would have been quite challenging to carry her over the massive logs.

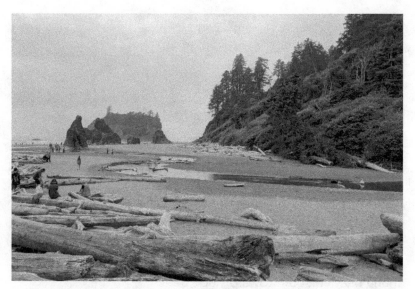

*Ruby Beach*

In the distance, there were several giant pieces of earth springing out of the ocean. The largest one, Abbey Island, is a beloved object of affection for photographers. Standing at over 100 feet in elevation, it almost always shows up in travel photos of the West Coast.

Beachgoers looked like tiny specks of dirt against the natural landscape of the beach. The only place I'd been that even came close to rivaling it was Redwood National Forest. It was humbling to feel so small standing there.

Ruby Beach gets its name from the reddish-colored sand that is sometimes visible along the shoreline. It didn't look red to me, but the view was breathtaking nonetheless.

The sand was much coarser than I imagined. Unlike the fine powder sand of Florida beaches that I'd grown up with on the Gulf coast, the sand at Ruby Beach varied in texture from large pieces of river gravel to that of fine rock salt.

The air was much cooler than Florida's tropical climate, too. Even in July, I had to bundle up in my fleece to avoid shivering. But it was still beautiful. By the time I reached the beach, the wind had picked up and I wished I'd brought my puff coat as well.

The sound of the water rushing against the shore was mesmerizing. Nature's calming energy was what I so desperately needed. Travel was, indeed, good medicine.

I watched as couples and families carefully stacked rock cairns together all along the beach, reminding me once again that I had no one to share the experience with.

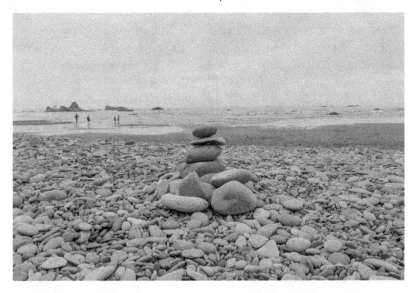

*Rock cairns on Ruby Beach*

I lingered for a moment, staring out at the vastness of the Pacific Ocean. As much as I wanted to blame my husband for the failure of our marriage, I knew he wasn't the only one to blame. In the cold ocean waves, I saw a reflection of myself. At some point in the relationship, I'd stopped being warm and loving. I'd turned cold and critical, and my unhappiness had almost certainly created more strain between us. I just hadn't been willing to see it.

Whether or not that contributed to the choices he made, it didn't really matter. He and I were on different paths now, and we'd been handed different lessons from the experience.

I considered walking further down the beach, but the idea of walking it alone made me sad. I found some dry rocks further up from the shoreline and sat down for a moment to rest, but they felt like ice cubes beneath me and I immediately stood up again. I decided to return to the van to have lunch overlooking the ocean instead. The climb back up the trail seemed further than it had coming down.

After returning to the van, I propped open the door and watched the bees collecting nectar from the bright pink foxglove blooms that lined the cliff just outside. As I gathered my lunch, I listened to the sound of the waves battering the shoreline below. It was relaxing, and I wished for a moment that I could just camp there for the night.

After I finished my lunch I was tempted to linger, but with the drive to the campground still quite a distance away, I wanted to leave enough time to get there before dark.

Ocean City State Park in Hoquiam, WA was much more my style than the RV park I'd stayed at the night before. With spacious campsites and a trail that led down to the beach, the minimalist amenities were barely even noticeable.

I settled into my campsite, which consisted of backing the van into the space and pulling the keys from the ignition, and then I quickly found my way to the trail that led out to the beach. I wanted to stretch my legs and do a little exploring before dusk, but because of the extra time I'd spent at Ruby Beach, I was cutting it close.

As I rounded the last corner down the path to the beach, I was greeted by a smattering of giant sand dunes, each one peppered with spiky mounds of grass. It reminded me of a camping trip that my husband and I had taken with friends several years back. We had set up our tent early in the evening, only to have it flooded out by heavy rains after dark, and we ended up sleeping in the car. I was sore for days afterward from sleeping in such an uncomfortably contorted position. I smiled at the memory, and felt even more grateful for my van.

There were only a few other people walking on the beach, but that was still quite a distance away. Other than that, I mostly had the beach to myself. I debated whether or not to walk all the way down to the water's edge, but decided to have a seat instead. I spotted a piece of driftwood in the sun and made my way over to it.

I slipped off my shoes and sank my feet into the warm sand. Maybe I had missed the sun more than I realized. Closing my eyes, I tilted my head back to feel the warmth of the sun on my face. My home in Issaquah had been nestled beneath enormous trees, and I was lucky to get three hours of sunlight a day at best, even in the height of summer. This felt glorious.

As the sun inched closer toward the horizon, I realized it was getting close to dusk. And I didn't like being out after dark. I felt vulnerable and I did my best not to call attention to the fact that I was traveling alone. I mostly stayed to myself at campgrounds, locking myself in the van early in the evening and avoiding conversations that might invite questions about my trip.

I'd at least thought to cover up the contents in the back of the van, by hanging a simple curtain, which I attached with magnets to both sides of the metal van interior.

I'd gotten used to strangers approaching me to ask questions about the van. At one campsite, an entire family approached me saying that they owned an RV but were enamored by the idea of van life. After I spent a few minutes answering the usual questions—whether it was gas or diesel, what kind of fuel mileage it got, and, of course, how much I'd paid for the van—one woman in the group took it one step further.

"What's behind the curtain?" she asked.

I was slightly shocked by the boldness of her question, but as time went on, that kind of questioning became more common. But still, it felt odd. To me, it was as if she'd marched onto my front porch and demanded to see the contents of a sock drawer in my bedroom.

"Just some camping gear," I said, hoping she would pick up on the subtle hint that she'd pried too far.

"Is that where your bed is? Can we see it?" she persisted.

"No, I'd rather not. I have a lot of my personal things in here." I said.

If pulling back the curtain wouldn't have exposed everything in the world that I owned, I might have been open to it.

But my reality wasn't the reality of most of the campers I met along the way.

I could tell she was disappointed, but thankfully she gave up.

After that, I decided to keep the van doors closed more often than I had before. It was still chilly outside even though the sun was out, so keeping the doors closed also helped keep the heat in.

In the morning, I sped through my morning routine and rearranged the contents of the van so I could get an early start to visit a friend who lived just south of the Oregon border. It was comforting to know that I had friends scattered throughout the country. For one thing, it made me feel more connected, which offered an added layer of security. But the further away from my Seattle network I traveled, the fewer friends I'd have to lean on if I needed help along the way.

After a lovely dinner at a local restaurant with my friend Dawna and her husband, I returned to their driveway, where I spent the night in the van. They'd invited me to stay inside for the night, but I felt more comfortable in the van. I didn't want to impose, especially during the busy work week. I didn't see the point in creating more laundry or upsetting their daily routines. But more than that, I'd already learned that if I wasn't sleeping in the van, I didn't sleep well out of fear that the van could be broken into.

Once again, temperatures dipped down into the 30s overnight, and I was thankful that I'd packed plenty of blankets. From time to time, I'd awaken to the sound of gravel shifting just outside the van, but I knew that it was probably an animal, since their property was situated on several acres in a rural area. Still, it was difficult to get used to the new noises with each new place that I camped.

From fireworks, to voices of other campers, to heavy rain, my brain spent a lot of time trying to determine if the sounds were innocuous, or a cause for concern.

The next morning, Dawna and I planned to go horseback riding at a nearby beach called Dibblee Point Park—except I was afraid of horses. They know they can do whatever they want with me because I have no idea what I'm doing.

In the small handful of times I'd been riding, my horse would almost always do the exact opposite thing I wanted it to do. I remember being on a group trail ride when I was little. My horse veered off the trail, marched me up the steep hillside, and tried to brush me off by riding close to random trees along the way.

So, when my horse-loving friend suggested a beach ride, I was a little apprehensive. But how could I not go? Horseback riding on the beach is something I'd never done before, and this trip was certain to include a series of things I'd never done before. That was the whole point, so I couldn't refuse.

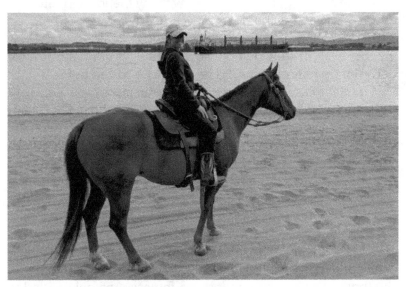

*Horseback riding at Dibblee Point Park*

The horse Dawna chose for me had a sweet, graceful demeanor, and I was relieved that, probably for the first time ever, I was able to relax in the saddle enough to actually enjoy the ride. The beach was quiet and calm, and I was thankful that I'd grabbed my wool fleece. The chilly breeze was brutal. But it was worth it.

When we returned to her home, we said our goodbyes and I turned the van south, toward Sunriver, OR, where I would visit with some more friends. Just like the previous night, I would spend the night in their driveway.

The drive to Sunriver was beautiful. I'd made the trip many times in the past few years, usually during the holidays. But the summer landscapes were equally as beautiful.

After an evening of laughter and recalling fun memories over a few glasses of wine, I made my way back out to the van for another night of driveway camping. Once again, I cocooned myself inside layers and layers of blankets. And I dreamed of warmer weather.

In the morning, I had breakfast with my friends and returned to the highway for the next leg of my adventure. As I moved further away from my safety net of friends, I realized that it was my first taste of truly being a solo traveler. If I ran into trouble between there and Texas, I'd have no one to call but AAA.

For that reason, I felt myself being even more cautious. I kept my fuel tank full, watched my tire pressure and gauges closely, and stayed hyper aware of everything and everyone around me.

Not long after crossing over into Oregon, I was running into some difficulties finding fuel. Standard diesel was becoming more difficult to find the further I ventured away from main interstates. Many gas stations carried 5% to 20% biodiesel blends, and I'd been advised not to exceed 5% by the Mercedes dealer. For that reason, I decided it would be smart to stay as close as possible to the major interstates, where truckers tended to congregate. Those stations almost always carried unblended diesel. The thought of being stranded in a remote area only added to my anxiety.

And then one afternoon my tire pressure warning light lit up on the dash. Temperatures had been steadily rising all day, and when the tire pressure exceeds 80 psi, there's an indicator light that issues a warning about potential traction control issues. I'd learned that already from a similar situation in the other van.

Knowing that I'd need to adjust the tire pressure soon, I pulled off the interstate and searched for a service station. As luck would have it, there was a tire center not far from the exit ramp. And after a quick pressure adjustment, I was back on the road. Being constantly on the move, it felt like there were a million tiny things to monitor.

By then, I was only four days into my trip, but I was quickly learning that driving conditions could change without warning. Rain, wind, temperature fluctuations, road conditions, elevation— every seemingly tiny shift in conditions resulted in completely different driving conditions. And from what I could tell so far, wind was the biggest factor. With the van's high roof, it didn't take much to blow me out of my driving lane. When the winds picked up, I'd have to grip the steering wheel tightly, especially when passing other high-profile vehicles.

# Driving in Circles

When I finally arrived at Crater Lake, I was immediately captivated by the deep blue color of the water. It was spectacular. I'd never seen water that color before.

Crater Lake is a famous caldera located in Oregon's Cascade Mountain range. The collapse of the Mount Mazama volcano created the crater-shaped hole that eventually filled in with snow and rain. It's now considered the deepest lake in the United States, at a depth of 2,000 feet.

I parked the van and walked to the overlook, where other tourists had gathered to take in the view. As I stood overlooking Wizard Island, the large landmass that is situated inside the cauldron-like lake, another wave of sadness hit me. Once again, I was surrounded by couples and families who were chatting, laughing, and taking photos together. And once again, I was alone.

I snapped a few quick photos and returned to the van to pull out my map. I still hadn't decided where to go next. Crater Lake was the last stop on my must-see list until Yosemite, and there were over 400 miles between them.

While I still experienced moments of sadness, solo traveling did have some perks. For one thing, I could go anywhere I wanted to without needing anyone else's input or agreement. And I could also stay as long as I wanted to when I got there.

But this would be my first night on the road without a clear destination. I hadn't made any camping reservations, and there were no more friends with driveways along my route.

I noticed on the map that Lake Tahoe was on the way to Yosemite, so I headed south toward Modoc National Forest. I hoped to run into a campground somewhere along the way.

As I drove deeper into California, the landscapes changed. The tall evergreens gradually gave way to thick layers of low-growing brush that covered the open fields like a blanket. The temperatures were much warmer than the brisk air I left back in Washington, too. It was a pleasant and welcome change.

The hum of the highway was addicting in a strange way. It distracted me from my new reality, putting me into a mellow trance.

I had hoped to reach Lake Tahoe before dusk, but my hopes were dwindling as I watched the sun inch closer to the horizon. I knew I'd be cutting it close. Really close. As I traversed the curvy roads leading into Incline Village, the sun kept sinking.

I came upon a couple of campgrounds along the way, but when I drove through them to scope them out, they were already full.

But by the time I reached Lake Tahoe, the sun had already set. The road was almost completely dark, and I did my best to dodge the hordes of people who walked precariously close to the shoulder that overlooked the lake. I had to keep driving. There were no turn offs or places to park.

Finally, I saw lights in the distance and felt a rush of excitement. I desperately needed a rest from driving, and I was hopeful to find a campground, or at least a small hotel. But as I drove into the city, it was buzzing with activity. Restaurant parking lots were completely full and there was still nowhere to pull off the road. I started to worry that I might not be able to find a place to park for the night.

I was nearing emotional meltdown level 3 status when I finally spotted a mostly empty parking lot at a casino. It was almost 10 p.m. by then, and I was on the verge of tears. I pulled the van into a spot and searched earnestly on my phone for a nearby hotel.

The thought crossed my mind that I could probably sleep right there in the parking lot. But I couldn't ignore the fact that it wasn't well lit, and there were a few other sketchy looking RVs parked nearby. My intuition begged me to reconsider, so

I continued searching. Finding no vacancies at nearby hotels online, I decided to call a few of them, just in case they held a few rooms back that weren't available online.

I breathed a sigh of relief when I was lucky enough to book the last available room at the Marriott South Lake Tahoe Resort. At $339.09, it was the most I'd spent so far for an overnight stay, but I was desperate to take a shower and sink my head into a soft pillow. I didn't even mind the idea of the air conditioner singing me to sleep. I just needed sleep.

From the sketchy casino parking lot, I steered the van back onto the road and through my droopy eyes, I did my best to dodge pedestrians while simultaneously searching for the hotel's entrance. But I couldn't find it. Each time I rounded the block where the entrance was supposed to be, I saw nothing to indicate an entrance. I took one right turn and was in California, and with the next right turn, I was in Nevada. I circled over and over again like the bald eagle back at Lake Sammamish. After the sixth time I rounded the block, I gave up and pulled into the same casino parking lot to call the hotel for directions.

By this time, I could no longer hold back the tears, and I imagined the poor woman who answered the phone must have been reconsidering her decision to book the room for me.

Why did everything have to be so hard? Why couldn't I catch a break? Why had I gone on this godforsaken trip in the first place? But those questions only brought more tears. And the answers didn't matter. The only thing that mattered was finding the entrance to the hotel. And by that point, I would have paid thousands of dollars to find it.

When I finally arrived at the hotel, I hesitantly handed over my keys to the valet. The van was too tall to fit into the parking garage, so I had to make arrangements at the front desk to have it parked near the front entrance. It made me uneasy knowing that someone else had my keys. Everything I owned was in that van, and I prayed the employees were trustworthy.

By the time I walked into my hotel room, it was almost 11 p.m., and I was too exhausted to shower. I kicked off my shoes, devoured a Clif bar, and fell facedown into the cold sheets, too tired to even care that I was still dressed in the clothes I'd been wearing all day.

Five hours later I found myself wide awake staring at the ceiling. My eyes were still swollen from my meltdown the night before, and I was still tired. But I knew that I needed to get on the road early if I had any hopes of making it to a campsite at Yosemite before dark. I didn't want to end up in the same predicament that I'd been in the night before. And I didn't like the fact that someone else had keys to my van.

After a much-needed shower and a couple cups of unimpressive hotel coffee, I felt slightly refreshed. I picked up my phone and noticed that my mom had tried calling several times. Still grumpy from the lack of sleep, I wasn't in the mood to chat. I also worried that she might misconstrue my tiredness for something else, and I didn't want her to worry. So, I texted her back with a quick update on my location and figured she'd call me back if it was something important.

I was genuinely grateful for friends and family members who called to check in on me occasionally, but I also genuinely wanted to be left alone. That was the constant internal struggle I battled with. I vacillated between feeling sad that I had no one to share all these amazing experiences with, and feeling grateful for my solitude. Grieving is messy. It's one of the reasons I'd chosen to go on the trip in the first place: to give myself space to grieve while I simultaneously figured out what to do with my life.

When the valet returned with my keys, I breathed a sigh of relief. When I saw that the van was still parked where I left it, I breathed another one. And when I found that the contents of the van seemed to have been left undisturbed, I finally relaxed.

# Yosemite

I continued south through the Hackamore region of California, and that's when I realized my little solo trip was real. By then I was far, far away from anyone I could call for help. I was on my own.

While I'd taken as many safety precautions as possible, like getting a AAA membership and doubling up on battery chargers, I felt vulnerable. As much as I wanted to believe that I was in complete control of my future, I knew that I wasn't. I was at the mercy of whatever the road held for me. The only thing I was doing was steering. And I was doing it alone.

But the aloneness felt bigger than the fact that I was rolling around in a van in the desert. I also felt alone in life. For most of my adult life, I'd been in a committed relationship. Being single was new to me. I was engaged before I was out of college, and now I was two divorces deep.

Being alone in the van was nothing; being alone in life is what scared me the most.

I'd been used to having a partner, someone to call if I needed help. But now there was no one to call. At that realization, I felt a wave of anger. I was angry that we'd tossed aside our wedding vows so easily. I was angry that we hadn't tried harder to repair the relationship.

But I was also angry at myself. I was angry that I'd given up a stable job in the midst of the unraveling. If I hadn't done that, I wouldn't be in this predicament, wondering how I was going to support myself financially, wondering where I would live, wondering how long I'd have health insurance. I chose to leave the safety of employment trusting that our marriage was salvageable, and that I'd have plenty of time to reestablish my career once I was emotionally ready. I wanted to blame him for all of it, but I knew that I only had myself to blame. It had been my choice, my doing.

But I'd have to sift through those realizations in my journal later. The only thing that mattered now was finding a campsite before dark.

The few hours of sleep I'd gotten the night before made me functional, but I was far from rested. When I saw the sign to the entrance of Yosemite National Park, I turned into the gas station on the corner.

After pulling the keys from the ignition, I leaned back in the driver's seat to stretch. My shoulders, which felt like they'd been carrying golf ball sized pieces of concrete for the past few days, lowered ever so slightly. Being stuck in the same position for hours and hours was rough. I had no idea how truck drivers did this for a living.

Since I'd reached my next stop ahead of schedule, I could feel the tension in my shoulders dissipating. My breathing slowed down, and I no longer felt anxious. In fact, everything seemed to slow down. Nature has always offered a cure for my anxiety.

Inside the gas station, I ordered a hamburger and fries from the café and returned to the van. I wanted to grab a quick lunch before driving further into the park. I also needed ice and wasn't sure if there would be any other stops along the way. As always, I wanted to be prepared.

But what I wasn't prepared for was just how beautiful Yosemite National Park would actually be. I'd heard people try to describe it. I'd seen photos. And I'd been to plenty of other beautiful parks, both in the U.S. and internationally, but there wasn't a picture in the world that could adequately capture Yosemite's beauty.

I meandered through the park's two-lane road behind a string of other park visitors. Every turn revealed a view equally as elegant as the last, and landscapes changed in an instant. There were lakes with stunning reflections of the enormous snow-covered mountains, trees as far as the eyes could see, open fields peppered with boulders and tall grasses, and waterfalls that threatened to take my breath away.

Even if it was possible to spend an entire lifetime there, I doubted it would be enough time to explore it all.

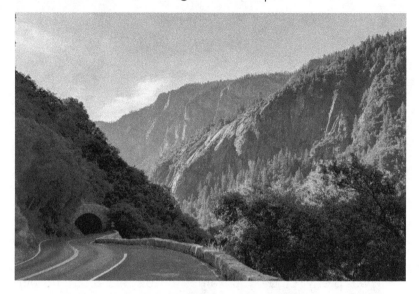

*View from a turnout at Yosemite National Park*

Periodically, I'd notice a turnout that had an open parking spot, and I'd promptly slam on my brakes to claim it. Outside the van it was chilly, and I had to put on my fleece every time I hopped out to snap a photo. But inside the van, the sunlight that beamed in through the windows warmed me as I drove.

It was still early in the afternoon when I stumbled upon the entrance to the Porcupine Flat campground, which was centrally located in the park. I decided to secure a site for the night, so I didn't have to worry about it later. Plus, I knew I'd be going to bed early. With the Lake Tahoe debacle still fresh in my mind, I realized the evenings were much more enjoyable when I settled into camp earlier in the day. That gave me plenty of time to relax, stretch, replenish my water supply, prepare dinner, shower, and prep my bedding before dusk. Not having to rush around made my life feel amazing.

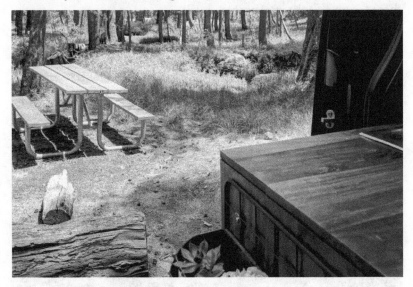

*Porcupine Flat Campground – Yosemite National Park, CA*

It was pretty standard for campsites to come equipped with a picnic table and charcoal grill, but this particular site also had a big metal box. Only a couple of times before had I camped at sites where bear boxes were necessary, and evidently, this particular campground was one of those.

Having just filled my cooler with ice, I somehow managed to slowly lower it to the ground and drag it by one handle over to the box, despite its heaviness. I pulled up the clip that secured it, opened the door, and slid the cooler inside. Next, I filled a grocery bag with the other food I had stored in the van, and added it to the metal box before securing the latch.

Afterward, I sat on the edge of the picnic table to take in the beautiful scenery around me. I felt calmer than I had back in Seattle. The sense of peace I felt gave me reassurance that I was making the right choice about leaving and replanting roots elsewhere. There were just too many familiar places and faces that triggered painful memories for me there.

It was still early, so there were only a couple of other campers in the park. I imagined most people were still exploring the trails and turnouts. I relished the silence. Behind my site, there was a small creek. The trickling water made me feel like I was sitting in a relaxation room at a spa.

A few minutes later, a ranger approached me. For a brief moment, I worried that I'd done something wrong. *Was I supposed to check in somewhere? Had I mistakenly chosen a site that was already reserved?*

"Hello," she said as she got closer.

I stood up from the picnic table and walked toward her.

"I just wanted to make sure you found the bear box," she said. "Please make sure you remove all food items—and I do mean all—from your van and secure it over there," she said, pointing to the box. "We've had a lot of trouble here recently. They know what grocery bags look like," she said.

We both laughed, and I immediately imagined Yogi bear and Boo Boo tapping on my van door in the middle of the night.

After preparing dinner, I visited the restroom one last time, and then locked myself in the van for the night.

Overnight temperatures were expected to be in the high 40s, almost 20 degrees warmer than it had been in Washington and Oregon, so I decided to crack the door windows slightly to allow for some air flow.

And I slept for 12 hours straight.

# Sequoia

The next morning, I felt more rested than I had in months. When I opened the door to the van, I was grateful to find that the chilly air wasn't as brutal as it had been for the past few days.

I was finally starting to feel grounded, which was ironic since I still had no roots. But I still felt a strong sense of peace that I hadn't felt for quite some time. My soul felt right.

There was nothing on my agenda for the day. No one to visit. No looming deadlines. Nowhere to be. Nothing to do. And for the first time since I was a kid, I was free to do whatever I wanted. The trip had finally served up what I was hoping for: space.

It felt so good that I considered staying there another night, but I was also eager to see more of the park. So I decided to move on after breakfast and find another campsite somewhere further down the road.

After learning my lesson in Lake Tahoe, I realized that I was going to have to do a better job of managing my time and energy. Six hours of driving a day was ideal, and eight hours of driving was my absolute max. I liked getting settled into my campsite by around 3 p.m. when possible. That gave me enough time to shower and prepare dinner before dusk.

I gathered my cooler and food supplies from the bear box and headed south on Big Oak Flat Road, where I made a quick stop at Bridalveil Fall. From the parking lot, I found a short, half-mile, round-trip trail that led back to the waterfall. From a safety standpoint, I hadn't felt comfortable hiking alone on any of the longer trails, so I wanted to take advantage of this opportunity.

When I got to the end of the trail, I stood still for a moment and stared up at the falling water. I chuckled to myself as I recalled its name—Bridalveil. It earned its name because of the way it sways back and forth in the wind, just like a bride's veil. It made me think back to both of my wedding days, never once imagining that either relationship would come to an end. But they did.

I knew it was going to take some time to unravel the complex lessons and takeaways from both of my marriages. But now that I had nothing but time on my hands, I'd be able to start making some sense of it all.

By the time I got back to the van, the parking lot was almost full. I was glad I'd gotten there early and hoped traffic wouldn't be too backed up on the main road.

The next stop on my list was Sequoia National Park, which I'd added to my bucket list after visiting the tallest trees at Redwood National Park a few years earlier. Now it was time to see the widest ones.

The van throttled loudly as I ascended the steep incline toward the park. From what I could tell, the engine temp was registering hot AF, so I quickly found a turnout and decided to rest for a few minutes. Breaking down in the middle of a national forest didn't seem like a good idea. And, although the van hadn't given me any reason to believe it wouldn't make it, I figured a small break wouldn't hurt. Plus, it would be a good excuse to get out and stretch my legs.

The central California temperatures were warmer than I was used to. It had been quite some time since I'd experienced heat on that level. Moving from Austin to Seattle, I'd gone from one extreme to the other, and I imagined my body was trying to figure out what the hell was happening.

When I arrived at the park visitor's center and flashed my magic annual pass at the entrance, I pulled into an open spot in the parking lot. As soon as I stepped out of the van, I couldn't help but turn my gaze upward. I remembered how small I felt years earlier when I was standing beneath the towering

Redwoods. It was humbling. My problems felt smaller. And that's the same way I was feeling again beneath the Sequoias.

I followed a few other tourists to a paved trail that led through Grant's Grove of giant trees. Some visitors snapped pictures of one another in front of the giant trees; others admired them from benches that were scattered along the shaded path. And then there was me, wandering alone down the trail.

It felt odd to be checking off so many bucket list items alone. I missed being able to talk with someone about what I was feeling and experiencing, laugh about the funny things we'd seen or heard, and share a meal at the end of the day.

But I also understood, at least on some level, that the solo trip was a necessary part of my healing. It was an adventurous act of self-care, a quest for understanding and acceptance. It was about learning to let go of the people and things that no longer belonged in my life. It was about coming to the realization that when someone wants to leave, I need to let them. The journey itself was a blank canvas on which I would be able to reimagine my life. I just had to figure out what I wanted my new life to look like.

After snapping a few pictures of the famous General Grant Tree, which stands roughly at 29 feet wide and 267 feet tall, I headed back toward the van to decide where to go next.

I pulled out my road atlas and scanned it to see if there were any nearby points of interest that I might like to visit. I'd grown to love my paper atlas. At first, it was nothing more than a "just in case" backup measure. If something happened to my phone, or if I didn't have access to the internet, at least I wouldn't get lost.

While I primarily used Google maps for navigation, I also loved having a big picture view of my options. With the paper atlas, I didn't have to zoom in and out on the small screen of my phone, and I could easily highlight the roads I'd already traveled. Maybe it's the same reason I prefer paper planners over digital ones.

I considered looking for a campground near the giant trees, but there really wasn't anything else that I wanted to see until the Grand Canyon, so it didn't make sense for me to linger.

The further south I moved, the higher the temperatures were climbing. During the day, temps were already reaching well over 100 degrees, and I was worried that overnight temperatures might be unbearable. Plus, I needed to do some laundry, so staying in a hotel would solve both of those issues.

With the Grand Canyon as my next destination, I decided to head toward Bakersfield, which was close to the next major highway turnoff, I-40.

On the second day of my trip, I began posting a few pictures of my travels on social media. For safety reasons, I was careful to only post photos of places I'd been the previous day. I didn't like the idea of anyone knowing exactly where I was at any given time.

I was surprised by how many other women—some I'd never even met—began messaging me. They shared words of encouragement about my journey. They shared personal stories that were similar to mine. And they also had a lot of questions about van life. Some wanted to know how I'd made the decision to leave my marriage. Others said they wished they had the courage to do a similar trip across the country. And some just wanted to send me good energy as I set out to rebuild my life.

I wasn't expecting that. I honestly didn't think my trip would affect anyone but me. But it had. And it was.

By that point, I'd traveled almost 1,600 miles since the morning I left on the ferry a week prior. It was the farthest I'd ever traveled alone. And it was the most alone I'd ever felt. But it also felt liberating. I felt more confident about my ability to do it because I had, indeed, done it.

When I got to my hotel in Bakersfield, I checked in and immediately gathered my clothes to do a load of laundry. The hotel didn't seem busy, but I noticed a lot of big work trucks in the parking lot when I arrived. There was only one other person in the laundry room, so I claimed the only open washer and tossed in my dirty clothes. I didn't even bother to separate them. I slid a few coins into the slot, poured in some detergent, pressed the button to start the machine, and returned to my room.

Later, on my walk back to the laundry room to move my clothes to the dryer, I thought back to how convenient it was having a washer and dryer at home. I was certain that if I did choose to live in the van full time that I'd be able to streamline some of my day to day routines, but the life of a nomad was anything but efficient.

The temperature outside had cooled off, and it felt nice even though I was in the middle of the desert. I probably could have camped in the van if I'd been gutsy enough to boondock, but then I wouldn't have been able to do my laundry. Everything was a trade-off.

After dinner, I returned to the laundry room to pull my clothes from the dryer, only to discover that several of my shirts and a pair of shorts were completely covered in grease. Then I thought back to the work trucks I'd seen in the parking lot on my way in. I tossed the ruined clothes into the garbage and loaded the rest of my clothes into my laundry bag.

When I got back to my room, I pulled out my atlas to retrace my steps from the day, and I realized I'd made a huge mistake. I thought I'd checked seeing the largest tree in the world off my bucket list, but I realized that I'd gotten it wrong. The General Grant Tree is the second largest, which meant that I totally missed seeing the General Sherman Tree, which was 29 miles further down the road. It didn't make sense to turn back. I'd have to see it some other time.

# Dust

The next morning before I checked out, I headed down to the lobby for some coffee and a quick breakfast. A couple of men were eating alone at separate tables, periodically glancing up at the TV that was mounted in the corner. I almost choked on my bagel when I heard the reporter say that someone had been stabbed to death overnight in a hotel parking lot just a few blocks away. And people say camping is dangerous. I was glad I hadn't decided to boondock.

My original plan was to head to the Grand Canyon next, but the thought crossed my mind that I might want to stop in Palm Springs on the way through. I'd heard from friends that it was beautiful, and the idea of spending some time at a spa didn't sound awful. If I did that, I could also hit Joshua Tree National Park. I'd already visited Los Angeles and San Diego before, so my other options were to continue driving south toward the Salton Sea.

But no matter which direction I went, the heat was going to be a factor. With no air conditioning in the van, at least when it wasn't running, I'd be forced to leave the windows down overnight for ventilation. And that felt a bit unsettling; it was just slightly above my risk tolerance.

After breakfast, I went with my original plan and plugged the Grand Canyon into my Google map. From Bakersfield to the Grand Canyon, I drove the entire 400-mile stretch in complete silence. No radio. No phone conversations. No phone calls. Nothing. Just the vibration of the diesel engine.

I'd never driven through a desert before. Sure, I'd seen the dry, sun-scorched earth from above when flying into Las Vegas, but I'd never really spent any time there. It felt ominous. Desolate. I noticed some giant dust clouds rising up in the distance, and for a moment I felt like Furiosa from *Mad Max: Fury Road* getting ready to ride through a sandstorm. It was just me and a handful of 18-wheelers on the highway.

I continued to receive messages from friends who'd been following my journey on social media, asking if I'd like to meet up somewhere along my route. I would have loved to have seen them; except I never quite knew exactly where I was going to be on any given day. I rarely camped near big cities, so figuring out where to meet would have been a logistical nightmare.

Besides, this trip wasn't really so much a vacation as much as it was a passage into the next phase of my life. It offered a safe transition. It was a different kind of adventure, an opportunity to clear my head, a safe space to have emotional meltdowns, and make some serious decisions about my life.

When I arrived at the Grand Canyon entrance, I was immediately overcome with emotion and overwhelm. There were buses and maps and parking lots and signs, all pointing in different directions to various lookout points.

I had done exactly zero minutes of research before pulling into the parking lot that day. And it showed. Some people plan a trip like this many years in advance, mapping out each experience carefully. I, on the other hand, just wanted to gaze out into the hole in the ground like they did in *National Lampoon's Vacation,* and then move on to my next destination. A quick little peeksie is all I needed to check it off my list.

I pulled the van into an open spot at a grocery store parking lot and walked toward a bus stop, where there were several maps of the lookout points posted. I asked a couple that was waiting on a nearby bench if they knew where the best viewing location was, and how long until the next bus was expected. They said they'd heard some bad weather was passing over a few areas, but the south end was clear. The next bus wouldn't be arriving for another 20 minutes, so I thanked them and decided to take a chance and drive around to see if there was an easier viewing spot. I'd gotten used to exploring on my own, and I kind of liked it.

I followed a line of cars pointed in the direction of the canyon, hoping they knew something I didn't. As we crept slowly, I could see cars lined up on either side of the road near a sign with the words "South Rim" prominently displayed on it. And a little further ahead, there was an opening with an amazing view of the Grand Canyon. But there weren't any open spots to park.

When the traffic in front of me stopped, I snapped a few quick photos from my window. It wasn't optimal, as several cars were obscuring the view. But I wasn't sure I'd be able to get a better shot with the swarms of people all fighting for just a few parking spots.

There wasn't a place to turn around even if I did see an open spot, so I had to keep with the flow of traffic and hope there would be a turnaround ahead. And sure enough, there was. As I rounded the turn, I silently prayed there would be a place to pull into when I looped around. And sure enough, there was.

I eased the van off the road into the open parking spot, which was right at the edge of the overlook at Pipe Creek Vista. And when I slid open the side door, the view was absolutely gorgeous. The scene brought me back to Waimea Canyon on the Hawaiian island of Kauai, a place I'd visited many times, including during my honeymoon eight years prior. This giant hole in the ground felt familiar, and it reflected exactly how I felt: expansively empty, yet open and ready to receive whatever I was meant to along the way.

It was the first time I truly felt unattached to outcomes. Openness felt good.

The trip had begun as a practical means of conserving my resources, to avoid spending money unnecessarily while I decided what to do with my life as a newly single woman. It was a way to give myself the time and space to clear my head and make better decisions than I likely would have while I was caught in the frantic whirlwind of selling the house and filing for divorce.

I walked to the edge of the canyon and looked out into the vast rocky landscape. Dark storm clouds were closing in. Keenly aware that other people were also waiting to take in the view, I snapped some quick photos before returning to the van, so I could set my sights on finding a campsite for the night.

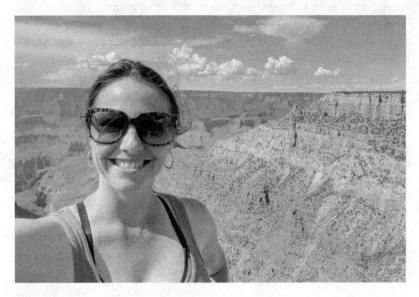

*Stacy at the Grand Canyon*

I was hoping to get settled in before the storm came. While the van didn't require much setup, I did need to refill my water containers and dump the gray water tank, and I preferred to do it when it wasn't raining.

When I arrived at the campground, I went through my usual checklist. First, I stopped at the front entrance. Some camp-grounds have a gated entrance, where you hand your payment to a park ranger, and others use a self-service pay station, where you select your site and then place your payment in an enve-lope, which goes into a lock box. This campground used the latter system.

I grabbed an envelope from the kiosk and proceeded to the loop of the campground. I liked to get a feel for the place before selecting a site, so I'd make some mental notes of the following as I drove: where the trash and gray water dump areas were, how many campsites were occupied, how clean the park was in general, which campsites were currently open, and how far away from the bathrooms they were.

Doing a quick drive-through also allowed me to do an intuition check. While it hadn't happened on this trip, in Europe it happened several times. We'd drive through a campground and for whatever reason, we just didn't have a good feeling about it, so we kept driving.

I usually liked to drive through the entire campground, but with the weather closing in, I knew I'd have to make a quick decision. It had already started to rain a little, so when I spotted a spacious pull-through site that was situated not far from the entrance, I pulled in and claimed it. I marked the site number on my envelope, tore off the stub that gets clipped to the post in front of the campsite, and jogged back to the front entrance to drop the envelope with payment in the lock box.

The rain was getting heavier, so I hurried back to the van, opened the sink cabinet, and grabbed the two 5-gallon water containers that needed to be refilled. It was much easier to carry two full containers than one because of the weight distribution. After filling both containers, I awkwardly wobbled back to the van, secured the water jugs beneath the sink, and headed toward the bathrooms.

I'd learned to scope out campground amenities in advance, so I knew what I had to work with. Some bathrooms were cleaner than others, some required special coins for hot water, and some only had basic amenities. Seeing no wall plugs or showers at this particular site, I decided that dry shampoo and Neutrogena cleansing wipes would have to do.

I jogged back to the van and locked myself inside. It was only about 4 p.m., but having been stuck in traffic at the Grand Canyon, I'd only had a bag of popcorn since breakfast and I was hungry. Unsure of how long the rain would last, I opted to make a peanut butter and jelly sandwich with fresh fruit for an early dinner. That way, I wouldn't have to drag out the camp stove in the rain.

Soon, the rain subsided, and I opened the sliding door of the van for some ventilation. Temperatures were in the upper 50s, which felt absolutely lovely. I pulled out my road atlas, my journal, and my box of books and settled in comfortably on the floor.

I read a few of my previously highlighted passages from *No Mud, No Lotus* and *Loving What Is*. They always seemed to help me shift my perspective whenever I got lost in painful memories. I'd been coming to the slow realization that there is indeed an art to suffering.

By that point, living the life of a nomad no longer seemed as difficult as it had been in the early days. I'd created some routines and had gotten more efficient with various tasks, from brewing coffee to showering. Life felt simpler and easier.

In the middle of the night, I awoke to the sound of more rain—and this time thunder. Then, I heard a strange tapping noise on the roof of the van, which I imagined was either hail or some small twigs or branches falling from the trees overhanging my site.

My thoughts drifted back to Zoey, and the fact that she wouldn't have liked having to pee in the rain. I wondered if she would have even enjoyed this little van trip.

Once again, I felt grateful to be locked inside my safe metal shell rather than outside in a tent. Van camping did have some serious advantages.

# Four Corners

The next day, I secured the van for travel and set my sights on the Four Corners Monument. On the map it looked like it was in a fairly desolate area, and I hadn't quite decided where to camp for the night. Some days I zeroed in on where I wanted to camp early in the day, but that morning I just figured I'd decide on the fly.

Somewhere along my travels I'd become enamored by the band Still Corners. Their album *Slow Air* is basically a story about leaving a relationship that ended abruptly, and then hitting the open highway—something I happened to know a thing or two about. But the song that really spoke to my soul was from one of their earlier albums *Strange Pleasures*, called "The Trip." In many ways, my journey—my trip—truly was the only thing keeping my soul alive. It was the only thing that brought me joy.

I hadn't realized how important it was to have something to look forward to. When life feels heavy and turned upside down, it's easy to feel overwhelmed. And I hadn't realized this adventure would be the difference between finding the energy to get out of bed in the morning and lying there wondering why I should bother.

When I thought about what I might experience on the road, I felt a sense of excitement. It fueled me in a way that my safe and familiar routines never could. And I realized that not knowing what lay ahead of me was part of what kept me driving on.

Noticing that my fuel gauge was approaching half a tank, I found my way to the nearest exit ramp for a top off. But I also braced myself for the inevitable. Getting out of the van almost always invited comments and questions from strangers. There were three common ones and the exchange generally went something like this:

Stranger: "How do you drive that big thing?"

Me: I'd flash a simple smile, but in my mind I'd say, "The same way you drive your Ford Festiva."

Stranger: "Is that a diesel?"

Me: "Yes."

Stranger: "What kind of mileage do you get?"

Me: "About 18."

That last question always caught people off guard, especially RVers who are lucky to get half that. With my large tank, I also have a range of about 500 miles, which is a nice bonus when you're traveling through remote areas where gas stations are few and far between. Sure, it's bigger but it isn't much different than driving a minivan. Just like anything, you figure it out eventually.

But the van did present a few challenges. For one thing, the diesel exhaust system was known to be temperamental. After hearing horror stories from other van owners in various online forums, I decided to never let the fluid drop below the half mark. But that required some planning.

Noticing that the DEF was nearing the halfway mark, I searched for the nearest Mercedes-Benz dealership on my Google map. There was one in Flagstaff, AZ, which was about an hour away. My plan was to dip down to Flagstaff, get the fluid topped off, and then jump back on the highway to hit the Four Corners Monument. It was a little out of the way, but I figured it wouldn't hurt to have a mechanic lay eyes on the van just in case something else needed attention. I was in and out of the dealership and back on the road in less than an hour.

But the trip to the monument took a lot longer than I expected. The winding road seemed to never end, and it was extremely hot, even for someone like me who loved feeling warm.

At one point I honestly thought I was hallucinating. I thought I saw a tiny, doll-sized person standing up in the middle of the road in front of me. I blinked several times, trying to determine if it was a stuffed animal or a real person. Had I been driving too long? For a moment, I swear whatever it was had its hand over its eyes scanning out over the horizon. Then, in a burst of energy, it scurried off the road just before the van rolled by. It was my first ever meerkat sighting.

When I finally reached the Four Corners Monument, I was tired of driving and desperately needed to stretch. I was glad I'd made the trip, but doubted I'd ever have a reason to come back again. And I wasn't excited about the long trip back through the desert at all.

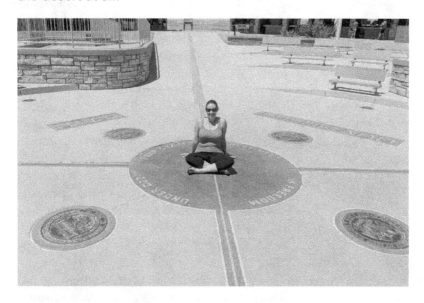

*Stacy at the Four Corners Monument*

When I arrived at the famous monument, there was a long line of people already queued up in the photo-opp line. Fortunately, it moved quickly, and I only had to wait about thirty minutes to strike my pose. I asked a stranger if she minded snapping a picture of me sitting on the spot that supposedly marks the convergence of the four states of Utah, Arizona, Colorado, and New Mexico. In hindsight, I may have made a poor choice on where the x marked the spot, but either way I got to check it off my bucket list.

On the walk back to the van I spotted a sign in the parking lot for fry bread. I immediately needed some. As far as I could tell from my drive in, there weren't many options for food in the area. I hadn't passed any restaurants or grocery stores, and the last time I'd been to a grocery store was back in California, so I didn't have a lot of food options.

I placed my order at the window of the food truck and the lady inside handed me a buttery, cinnamony slice of heaven. It was ridiculously good. One of the things I love about traveling is getting to sample different foods in different regions, especially when traveling internationally. But on this trip, I hadn't dined out much since I'd left on the ferry.

With the exception of having dinner with my friend and her husband in Oregon, and the burger I'd picked up on my way through Yosemite, I'd managed to prepare the majority of my meals in the van. I preferred it that way. It was more affordable. And since most of the campgrounds weren't near grocery stores or restaurants, it just made more sense from a practical standpoint.

I popped the last bite of fry bread into my mouth and hopped back in the van. I decided to follow the I-40 corridor eastward, so I needed to head south from there. Knowing how long the drive had seemed on the way in, I decided to take another route into Albuquerque, NM, hoping it was more scenic, or at the very least, different.

My hope was to find a campground just outside the city, but I realized about an hour into my drive that I was dangerously close to repeating my Lake Tahoe mistake. My Google map arrival time kept getting later with each stoplight I sat through, delaying my arrival in Albuquerque by a few minutes each time.

# A Bum in the Driveway

By the time I finally reached Albuquerque, it was already 4 p.m., well after I liked to be getting settled into my campground for the night. But I was drooling over the thought of crispy, fresh vegetables. Life on the road left me with limited options when it came to produce. My cooler of ice didn't last long, which meant it was more difficult to keep fresh fruits and vegetables on hand, especially in the desert's brutal heat. A few times, I'd opened the lid to find water-logged food bobbing in a pool of lukewarm water. Peanut butter and jelly became a dependable staple when all else failed.

After driving all day, and only snacking on fry bread, I needed something more substantial. I located the nearest grocery store on my map, a Whole Foods, where I planned to grab a quick salad and search for a campsite. But I hadn't realized how late it was. But the time I parked the van in the parking lot, the sun was already beginning to set. And since I hadn't showered the night before, I desperately needed to freshen up.

The closest campground I found was still an hour's drive away, and arriving that late meant it would be unlikely to find an open campsite.

While I ate my salad, I searched my map to see if there was a Planet Fitness nearby. I hadn't yet used my Black Card because I'd been traveling through such remote areas, but I was thinking that I might have to resort to boondocking if I couldn't come up with a better plan. And at minimum, I needed a shower.

But then it dawned on me that I might have another option. Kelly and Cassandra, some friends that I'd met back in Seattle, had recently moved to Albuquerque, so I messaged Kelly on Facebook to see if they minded having a hobo spend the night in their driveway. While I awaited Kelly's response, I continued on to the local Planet Fitness to get my shower out of the way.

When I checked my phone after showering, Kelly had responded to say they welcomed my hobo proposal. So, I plugged their address into my phone and steered the van their way. It was so great to exchange hugs and see some familiar faces. We visited for a few minutes outside the van, and then said our goodnights. In exchange, I promised to treat them to some French-pressed Seattle coffee in the morning.

As I settled in for the night, I realized it would be the first time since I'd been camping in the van that I didn't need a blanket. It was still hot after the sun went down, and I actually had to pull out a small battery-operated fan that had been tucked away in the back for the entire trip. I cracked the front windows of the van and then pointed the fan directly on me so I didn't lie there sweating all night.

The next morning, I treated my friends to some freshly pressed coffee that reminded us all of our beloved Seattle. As we sat sipping from our mugs in their living room, we shared stories and marveled at how mysteriously life often plays out. I thanked them again for giving me a safe place to spend the night, and I climbed back into the driver's seat of the van.

I briefly considered heading south toward El Paso, but the heat concerned me. While I was grateful to finally not have to shiver myself to sleep, sweating profusely through the night didn't exactly sound like a great alternative. Mid-July probably wasn't the best time of year to go exploring the desert, so I scratched that off my list.

I also considered going north, toward Mesa Verde. I'd never been to Colorado, and I was curious about Cliff Palace. I'd originally added it to my bucket list when I decided to do the van trip. It reminded me of Petra, except it was accessible by van.

# Texas

Ultimately, I decided to continue heading east toward Wichita Falls, TX, where my great-aunt lived. I'd already planned to visit Austin, and she was on the way. It had been at least ten years since I'd seen her at my grandfather's eightieth birthday gathering.

I texted my mom to see if she had any contact information for my great-aunt, and she sent two phone numbers. I called them both, but no one answered. So, I decided to show up on her doorstep unannounced and hope she was there. My great-aunt is a spunky woman in her early nineties who has a knack for storytelling. Her endearing nature easily captures the attention of anyone in her sphere. She tells it like it is, and she's captivating.

I arrived at her house, carefully double checked the address on my phone, and rang the doorbell. When she opened the door, I could tell she didn't recognize me.

When she finally did, she swung the door wide open and held out her arms to hug me. It felt so good to be near family again.

We spent the evening laughing, sharing stories, and laughing some more. I made a silent vow to myself that I would continue dropping in on friends and family unannounced, because life's just too short not to.

I woke up the next morning wondering how I would ever know when my trip was over. I'd only been on the road for ten days, but it already felt like months. And even when I did finally arrive at my mother's house in Florida, it wouldn't necessarily mean my trip was over. Florida was only a placeholder on the map.

The purpose of the trip was to give myself the space to figure out what to do next, but I hadn't really spent much time formulating a concrete plan. My days had been consumed by menial tasks, like finding a place to shower, locating a campsite, and filling water jugs. The trip had become a treasure hunt with no treasure in sight.

Slowly, I was becoming a vagabond.

I said goodbye to my great-aunt and turned south again toward Austin, a place I'd called home for six years before moving to Seattle.

When I rolled into town, I had one destination on my mind. For days, I'd been craving breakfast tacos. Torchy's Tacos are my absolute favorite—the Crossroads and the Trailer Park breakfast tacos simply cannot be rivaled.

After my dose of morning tacos, I gave myself a tour of the city, driving through familiar places and recalling the memories I'd made there.

I remembered how my husband and I spent almost every Friday night eating fajitas and drinking margaritas at Chuy's.

I remembered shopping at the Austin Farmers' Market nearly every Saturday morning.

I remembered spending fun nights out with friends on 6th Street.

Knowing that I'd be coming through town, I'd messaged some friends a few days before my arrival to let them know I'd be in the area, and hoping we'd be able to meet up for drinks. A handful of friends confirmed, and we planned to meet up later that night at The Domain, a shopping hub with a ton of restaurants and happy hour venues.

With no camping options in the city that I knew of, I decided to splurge and book a room at a local hotel. Temperatures during the day were approaching 100 degrees, so spending the night in the van didn't make much sense.

Several times along my trip I wished that I'd been able to somehow figure out how to have at least part of the van build-out completed before I left. Traveling would have been so much easier with a source of heat and air conditioning. I could do without a shower, but the harsh temperature swings were an absolute bitch.

After settling into my hotel room, I noticed how tired and haggard I looked when I saw myself in the mirror. Evidently, I needed more rest than I realized. I immediately called down to the front desk and booked another night's stay, and then booked a massage for the following morning at a spa that was within walking distance of the hotel.

Self-care was slightly more challenging from the road, but it wasn't impossible.

I'd covered a lot of ground in a short amount of time, and I wasn't even sure why I was moving so quickly. On average I'd driven 300+ miles a day. But there was no real sense of urgency. I was in no rush. I could have easily stayed two nights at some of the campgrounds earlier along my trip, so I had more time to explore. But I hadn't. Maybe I'd gotten so used to rushing around during the move, that it was just out of habit.

After meeting up with a few friends for drinks, I returned to my hotel room. I was more emotional than I'd expected. The friends I'd spent the evening with were mutual friends of both mine and my husband's, and each one of them had ties to a life that no longer belonged to me.

Even so, I was grateful that they'd been so willing to stay connected with me, even under the awkward circumstances. And I was equally grateful that none of them had asked about the details behind our split. The *why* didn't really matter anyway.

After my massage the next morning, I drove past the old house we lived in. I remembered the fun dinner parties we'd hosted, the Christmas decorations I used to put up in the living room, and all the landscaping I'd done in the back yard that the dogs had dug up within hours of it being planted. I laughed recalling some of the ridiculous moments.

Later that evening, I had dinner with a friend at one of my

favorite restaurants. It was nice to catch up, but I knew that I'd be ready to move on the next day.

As I tucked myself into the hotel sheets that night, I felt complete. In Austin, I'd checked off all my favorite restaurant menu items, visited with friends, and released that part of my life to the rest of my random memories.

# The Longest Leg

When I left the hotel the next morning, I knew I'd reached a turning point.

But it wasn't a good one.

I was no longer looking forward to anything on my trip. I still had at least 1,000 miles left to go, and nothing ahead of me felt exciting. There was nothing but the highway between where I was and my mother's driveway.

And the truth is, I didn't really want to go to Florida. Sure, I'd chosen it as an arbitrary end point when I boarded the ferry because I had family there, and I knew that I'd eventually want to stop to visit them. But since nothing else had materialized along my trip, part of me worried that I might end up there permanently.

I wasn't sure if my resistance to Florida was more about missing Seattle, or if I simply didn't like the idea of circling back to where I'd grown up. In some ways, the thought of living there again felt like moving backwards.

But as much as I didn't want to see it then, the truth was that Florida met my two biggest requirements: warmth and no snow. While the rest of my criteria could have easily be met in just about any medium-sized city in the U.S., Florida offered the added bonus of having access to over 600 miles of beaches.

But still, I'd hoped that I would have felt drawn to a place somewhere along the way like I did back in Issaquah. But so far nothing had beckoned me to stay longer than a day or two.

For every city that I envisioned myself living in, I came up with at least one reason to rule it out. I loved the history of Washington D.C., but I didn't like the harsh winters. I adored the al fresco California lifestyle, but I didn't really like the desert landscapes. I was quite fond of the Seattle and Austin food scenes, but I had too many memories tied to both.

There was something to dislike or worry about no matter where I imagined myself living: the Pacific Northwest's never-ending rain, tsunamis, earthquakes, volcanos, snowstorms, and fires; middle America's tornados, ice storms, dust storms, and droughts; and Florida's sinkholes, sharks, snakes, hurricanes, and gators. Every time I considered a potential new place to call home, I found a reason to cross it off my list.

And the truth was, I really did miss the Pacific Northwest, with its mossy, tree-lined landscapes, snow-capped mountains—and even the relentless rain. I'd grown to love the cooler weather, the gray days that were perfect for staying in and reading, and the genuinely kind people. I'd made some wonderful friends in the past couple of years there.

Several times throughout the trip, I fought the urge to turn the wheel around and head back to Washington State. It's where my heart wanted to be. It's where my home was, or at least used to be. But I kept driving. I needed to make a clear-headed decision about where to settle down.

I thought I'd be able to think clearly on the road, but so far it hadn't offered me as much space to think as I'd hoped. But if I was being honest with myself, I knew deep down that it was because I hadn't allowed myself the space. I could have easily slowed down my pace, or lingered at various stops along the way. But I kept moving, as if I was afraid of what I might discover if I really thought about what I wanted.

The air in East Texas felt sticky and steamy. I noticed a church sign near Paige, TX with the following message: *Satan called, he wants his weather back.* I imagined he did.

That night, I decided to stay at a Residence Inn near Baton Rouge, LA. While hotels were definitely more expensive than campgrounds, air conditioning was no longer negotiable.

The next morning, I crossed over to the Mississippi Welcome Center, where I was pleasantly surprised to find a free gray water station. The little things weren't so little on the road. Van life had made me appreciate the small conveniences a whole lot more.

Emptying the gray water container was an important task. If I let it go too long, it would smell absolutely horrible in the van. While I only used the sink to brush my teeth, do a few dishes, and wash my hands, it was enough to create a disgusting stench, especially as I'd moved into hotter climates.

After another full day of driving, I spent the night at a Courtyard Marriott in Duluth, GA, where vacuuming the hallways after 8 p.m. evidently wasn't frowned upon. Between the mosquitoes and the extreme heat, I went ahead and crossed it off my list of possible places to relocate.

Once again, I missed my home back in Issaquah. I missed drinking coffee on my wooden swing with my hummingbird friend. I missed the sound of rain on the trees. I missed so many things about my life there. But, oddly, I didn't miss my marriage. I hadn't realized just how unhappy I was until I felt the freedom of the road.

# Disturbed

After making another stop to visit with family in Spartanburg, SC, I was eager to get back on the road the next morning. I was anxious for some nature therapy and decided to look for a campground for the night. Having spent the last six nights in an actual bed, I was oddly missing the uncomfortable floor of the van. Or maybe I was missing the solitude.

I was still trying to find the right balance between solitude and connection. Sometimes I just wanted to be left the hell alone to grieve, and other times solitude brought on such strong emotions that connection was the only cure for my sadness.

I zeroed in on a national forest in North Carolina that was just a little over two hours away. The Carolinas were on my short list to explore as a possible place to relocate. Aside from the occasional winter storm, it was more temperate than other northern states, and also offered plenty of mountainous hiking trails.

I didn't know it at the time, but that would end up being the final night of my trip. And it was the only night of my 17-day adventure that I felt scared for my safety.

The Uwharrie (pronounced you-warr-ee) National Forest is just shy of 80 square miles in size, and it's the smallest national forest in the state.

The West Morris Campground isn't accessible near any major highway. I had to drive through a series of residential neighborhoods and large tracts of land before stumbling upon the entrance, almost by accident.

I pulled into the entrance of the campground and grabbed an envelope from the self-service pay station. The camping fee was only $5 for the night, the cheapest of any campground I'd been to since I owned the van.

As usual, I took a quick drive through the campground first to get a sense for how crowded it was, and whether or not it seemed clean and safe. I climbed back in the van and headed into the main loop of the park. I only noticed one other car at one of the first sites beyond the entrance. It was a woman and her dog, and she was setting up her tent.

I found an open site at the opposite end of the campground, just a few spots away from the restroom, and returned to the front entrance with my payment envelope.

Once I got settled into my spot, I made an easy dinner that didn't require the camp stove, and began preparing my bed for the night.

Then I heard the crunch of tires on gravel and saw a car pass by in front of the van, heading toward another campsite in the distance. A man and woman got out and appeared to be assessing whether they wanted that spot. Soon, they got back in the car and drove away.

It was still early, but I'd gotten used to turning in not long after the sun went down. Just before I closed the van door, I noticed the same car had returned, and the same couple as before was setting up camp and starting a fire.

At 1:19 a.m., I awoke to voices outside the van. To say that I was disturbed is putting it mildly.

West Morris Campground in Uwharrie National Forest

"A black Mercedes," said a man with a southern accent. A woman's voice mumbled something back to him that I couldn't quite make out.

When my eyes finally opened, I was immediately blinded by two flashlights beaming in through the windows. Thankfully, I'd drawn the cab curtain before I slipped into my sleeping bag, so they couldn't see me.

At first, I thought they were park rangers. At Yosemite, I was used to seeing rangers making rounds to ensure campers stored their food safely in bear boxes. But these were definitely not rangers.

The lights faded and the sound of crunching gravel underfoot intensified as they moved toward the back of the van. "It has Washington plates!" exclaimed the man. "That is just soooo strange," he added.

*Dude, you're the one snooping around a remote campground on a random Thursday night. Is that not strange?*

They made their way around to the front of the van again, and the flashlights returned.

"There's a 2018 road atlas!" he said, shining the light onto the passenger seat. "That is just weird."

*Who is this guy, Giorgio Tsoukalos?*

When the lights and voices finally faded, I peeked around the curtain and watched the flashlights dim into the darkness toward the campsite I'd seen the couple at earlier.

As I sat up trying to process what had just happened, I glanced up toward the window again and saw a single flashlight bobbing in the distance, moving toward me slowly.

But this time I was wide awake.

I crouched behind the passenger seat with the curtain drawn as I watched the man approach the van. He was wearing jeans and a t-shirt, and the flashlight he was carrying illuminated his round, stubbly cheeks, and dark, thinning hair.

"Is there something I can help you with?" I asked brusquely through the window, which was cracked ever so slightly for air circulation.

Startled, he jumped back, hobbling a little at first and then bursting into a fit of laughter. "Oh my God! Oh my God! You scared me!" he said as he continued laughing loudly. "It's just that this...this is a black Mercedes...with Washington plates," he said, still laughing hysterically.

"Yes?" I replied.

But he just stood there, staring at the van in silence.

"Have a good night," I said, hoping he would take it as an invitation to leave.

And he did.

I was relieved, but I couldn't go back to sleep. It was all so bizarre and unsettling that I knew I needed to leave, so I began searching for nearby hotels. Except when I looked up from my phone just a few seconds later, I saw the flashlight coming toward me again for a third time. But this time he was bolder, tapping on the van door when he arrived.

"Is there something you need?" I asked gruffly. I was beyond pissed.

"I'm sorry. It's just that this is a black van out here...a Mercedes...and it has Washington plates...you just scared me," he said.

"Well, you scared me when you came here at 1:19 a.m. shining your flashlights in my window," I said.

He laughed.

I didn't.

"I'm sorry, I didn't mean to bother you," he said as he turned and left. But by that time, I had my shoes on and the keys to the van in my hand, contemplating my exit strategy.

I considered briefly whether he might be under the influence of something, or mentally unstable. But I knew that it didn't really matter in the grander scheme of things. It was time for me to go. I still hadn't been able to find a hotel in the area, but I did find a rest area. The closest one was still a 30-minute drive, which wasn't optimal, but it would have to do.

But just as I was about to crawl into the driver's seat to start the engine, I noticed that he was headed back again, for what would be the fourth time in less than an hour. This time he knocked even louder on the passenger door.

*The SOB was getting bolder.*

"Well, hello again," I said, not at all trying to disguise my disgust at his intrusion.

"Hey, I'm sorry," he said. "I just wanted to apologize."

"You've done that already," I blurted out.

"It's just that this van...out here..." his voice trailed off as he broke into laughter again.

I said nothing.

Finally, he turned to leave just as quickly as he arrived, but

I was ready this time. I waited until he got halfway back to his campsite before I slid into the driver's seat, lowered the emergency brake, started the engine, and popped the van into drive. I cranked the wheel to the left—in the opposite direction of Weirdy-McRound Cheeks, and hit the gas.

As I drove toward the exit, I prayed that the gate would be unlocked when I got there. At some campgrounds they lock the entrance at night for safety reasons, an amusing irony given my current situation. I remembered reading on the website that this was one of those campgrounds, and I wasn't exactly sure what I'd do if I got there and found that the gate was locked. That would put a major hiccup in my egress plan.

I briefly ran through some possible scenarios as I drove. Would I drive straight through the gate? How badly would it damage the van? How long would it take for 911 to dispatch someone if things turned even weirder?

As I rounded the final corner of the campground loop, I exhaled a sigh of relief when I saw that the gate was wide open. I hit the gas, glancing every few seconds in the rearview mirror to make sure there were no headlights behind me.

For miles I drove in darkness, swerving around snakes stretched out across the road, and dodging dozens of deer who were clearly annoyed by the disruption.

When I saw that there were still no headlights behind me, I relaxed a little, but I was still trembling. Tears filled my eyes and an extreme sense of gratitude washed over me. I was grateful that I'd been locked safely inside the van rather than outside in a tent. I was grateful that I'd chosen to buy a van instead of a pull-behind camper, since I didn't have to get anything road-ready. All I had to do was crank the key and roll. And I was grateful that I'd had the foresight to back into the parking space rather than pull in, making my exit even easier.

I smiled, imagining the man scurrying back to his campsite when he heard the strange van-spaceship start up behind him. I mean, had he seriously never seen a Sprinter van before? What was so strange about a campervan at a campground? I was exhausted and still half asleep.

At some point on the way to the rest stop, I missed a turn and had to backtrack for a short stretch. By then, my adrenaline had worn off and I was feeling more annoyed about my sleep being interrupted.

I imagined this is how many boondockers feel when they get the 2 a.m. knock. I value my sleep too much for that.

When I finally saw the bright blue glow of the Rest Area sign, I was relieved. And I felt even better when I saw a few cars parked in the parking lot. But I was still on high alert.

Still exhausted, I locked the van and returned to my sleeping pad in the back of the van, which was exactly where I'd left it.

It was my 16th night on the road since I'd left on the ferry, and that felt like a million years ago.

The trip wasn't fun anymore.

# PART III:
## Manifest

# The Sunporch

After a couple hours of sleep at the rest stop, I decided to get the last leg of my trip over with. The drive to my mother's house would take roughly ten hours with stops—more than my usual eight- to ten-hour limit—but I was ready for the trip to be over.

With the lack of sleep, I was feeling grumpy. I was disappointed that I hadn't felt as transformed by the trip as I'd hoped. I hadn't discovered any viable places to settle down along the way, and I felt like a lost soul. But beyond that, I was frustrated that I hadn't given myself more time to grieve the end of my marriage. I was disheartened that I was beginning the next chapter of my life, yet I still had no clear plan for my future.

Exactly six weeks prior, I'd rolled down my driveway in Issaquah for the last time, feeling hopeful about my future. And for the past seventeen days, I'd been wandering aimlessly across the country on a vision quest to figure out what to do next. My possibilities were endless. But here I was now, facing the reality that I was just a stinky bum with greasy hair driving to my mommy's house.

I sat with my negative thoughts while I listened to the monotonous hum of my wheels on the highway. It hadn't been the trip I'd envisioned.

In my Candy Land mind, I'd expected the trip to bring me clarity, to offer up a clear plan for my future. I'd expected to have come to terms with the end of my marriage and filed it away neatly in my "lessons learned" file. I'd expected an earth-shattering spiritual transformation, but none of that had happened.

I laughed out loud when I realized that a little over two weeks was a pretty tall order to get my shit together. Perhaps I'd been slightly unrealistic in my expectations. Decisions—especially life-changing ones—take as long as they take. And grieving takes as long as it takes, too.

When I pulled into my mother's driveway, I was greeted by familiar smiling faces—my mother, stepfather, and grandmother were standing on the front porch waving. I flashed back a forced smile as I put the van in park and turned off the engine, secretly wishing I had a few more minutes alone to gather my composure.

I hadn't showered in two days, and I was physically and emotionally exhausted. Part of me wasn't ready for the trip to be over, but another part knew there was nowhere left to go. I'd practically driven from one corner of the U.S. to the other in just seventeen days.

But I couldn't run away from my reality any longer; it was time to make some decisions about my future.

For the next seven nights, I slept on a fold-out cot on my mom's sunporch. I felt unsettled, sitting with the heartbreaking reality that my trip hadn't brought the clarity I'd hoped for. It left me, once again, with nothing to look forward to.

That first week, I spent my days feeling anxious about not having a plan for my future, and my evenings feeling guilty about the fact that I was a forty-something adult still living with her mother. At this stage of my life, I was supposed to have my shit together, and it was beginning to wear on me.

I doubled down, devoting extra time to my morning self-care practice. I spent hours journaling, studying *A Course in Miracles*, and doing my best to take inventory of my options. But there were just too many options. Being able to go anywhere and do anything felt overwhelming.

While I was grateful that my mother and stepfather had opened their home to me, I was eager to have my own space.

I considered renting a long-term spot at an RV park, but since the van didn't have air-conditioning, it just wasn't realistic.

Temperatures were climbing to well over 100 degrees inside the van after sitting in the sun for just a few minutes. Florida sunshine is beautiful, but it's also brutal. Living in the van just wasn't an option.

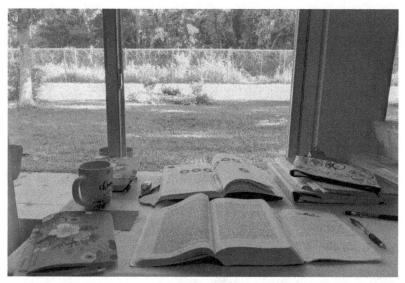

*Stacy's morning self-care practice on the sunporch*

And besides, I'd learned that life on the road wasn't exactly the calming, spiritual experience that I'd hoped for. I was constantly moving and there was little time for stillness.

I also considered renting a small studio apartment somewhere, but wasn't keen on the idea of signing a year-long lease. I didn't know exactly where I wanted to be, and I didn't want to get locked into anything long term, for the very same reasons I hadn't wanted to rent a place in Seattle.

But my biggest fear was that I'd have to settle for something that didn't light my soul on fire. I'd already done that too many times. And it never ended well. I always eventually found myself seeking an escape.

When I wasn't journaling, I went for walks alone at nearby parks. I spent time at the gym. And I enjoyed spending time with my family, something I hadn't done in many years.

But one morning I woke up with a clear vision of what I needed to do.

More than two weeks of driving had given me some new perspective, but it hadn't given me the space that I'd hoped for. I needed my own place to relax, a place to sort out everything that had happened, a place to grieve properly, and a place to lay my head that didn't involve having to find a new place to park every day.

After easing myself off the cot in the sunroom and pouring myself a cup of coffee, I joined my mother and stepfather in the living room.

"I know what I need to do next," I said.

Simultaneously, they leaned back and placed their coffee cups on the table next to the couch, clearly bracing themselves for what I was about to say.

"I'm going to the beach," I said.

Except it wasn't just some fleeting desire to book a room at a hotel so I could run my toes through the sand. It was a command that had been issued from somewhere within my soul. I didn't just want to go to the beach. I *needed* to be there. I didn't know why exactly, but one way or another, I was going.

# Manifesting

Some people are goal setters, and some people are manifestors.
I used to be a goal setter.

But goals are rigid and concrete.

That's why when you fall short of your specific, measurable,
attainable, realistic, and time-bound SMART goals, you almost
always feel like there's something wrong with you. And it's coun-
terproductive, because with every failed goal, you believe a little
less in your abilities to change anything about your life. Goals
are unforgiving—either you achieve them, or you don't.

Manifesting, on the other hand, is unlimited.

When it comes to manifesting, the first step is to get clear
about what you want. And I mean crystal clear—to the point
that you can see it, taste it, and feel it. Manifesting is a sensory
experience. And, yes, at first it feels woo-woo AF.

The second step to manifesting is actually counterintuitive to
the goal-setting process. In order to manifest, you have to stay
open. Not only do you have to stay open to the process of how
it unfolds, but you also have to stay open to the outcome itself.
Because sometimes the outcome is better than you envisioned,
and if you limit yourself to just what you believe is possible, you
might miss out on so much more.

Manifesting isn't passive. It still requires planning and action.
Once you've gotten clear about what you want, you still have to
do the work to get it. Sometimes your investment of time and

energy is less than what you expected, and sometimes more. You have to be willing to show up for your dreams.

Manifesting isn't forcing, either. It doesn't require you to bulldoze your way through obstacles at the expense of other people's joy.

I spent the morning scouring the internet for beach rentals, most of which were about two hours away from my mom's house. I'd grown up in the area, so I knew the Gulf coast beaches fairly well, and it didn't take long for me to pinpoint where I wanted to be—down to the exact building.

I found a couple of vacant units that were available and left a few messages with listing agents, hoping I'd be able to schedule a trip down later in the week.

The plans were set in motion.

But then something happened that I wasn't expecting. And that's how I know it was manifested. Later that day, my aunt and uncle came over for dinner, and I casually mentioned to them that I was looking to rent a condo on the beach.

"I'm not sure exactly where it is, but our friend has a rental somewhere over there," my aunt said. "In fact, I think he's looking for a tenant right now."

*Wait, what? There's no possible way it could be anywhere near the area I had been looking at. Or could it?*

Before I realized it, my aunt was texting her friend for the address of his condo. And it turns out that it wasn't just near the area I was looking, but it was in the exact building that I had already decided I wanted to be in.

*Manifested.*

The vision that I woke up with on a random morning led me to exactly where I was supposed to be.

I manifested the eff out of that condo, and it proved to me that it's possible to manifest anything when we get clear enough about what we want. And once we do get clear, once we set the wheels in motion, it almost always happens more quickly than we expect. Because if you don't ask, you don't get.

And here's the thing: You are always manifesting. Whether you realize it or not, you are manifesting something right now.

You know those feelings you get? Those hunches, tingles, and chill bumps? Those are signals for you to pay attention. If I hadn't followed my intuition when I got the nudge to go to the beach, I might still be sleeping on a fold-out cot today. If I hadn't spoken my desire out loud when my aunt and uncle were visiting, I might have ended up somewhere else entirely.

I don't think I fully understood until that moment that we manifest everything we experience in life.

In fact, if I was really honest about it, I had to accept that I had manifested the end of my marriage as well. Deep down, I didn't believe we were going to make it. I constantly waited for the other shoe to drop. I expected dishonesty. I expected the worst. And that's exactly what I got. I manifested the whole thing. Because our reality is deeply rooted in what we think about and what we believe.

# Water

I arranged to see the condo that my aunt and uncle's friend owned the following week. My mom and I drove down together and had lunch on the beach before heading over to the condo. I was fairly certain it was the one, but I needed to see the space before signing the contract. I mean, how could any view of the beach be disappointing?

As soon as the door opened, I saw it. The aqua blue water was all I could focus on. The rest of the unit no longer mattered. It was clean and tidy and that was enough for me. The view alone was worth the price of rent. With direct access to the beach, a pool, and laundry facilities on site, I felt like I'd hit the lottery. This is where my soul had been leading me. And I'd followed it, even if I'd done so begrudgingly at times.

It was the perfect space for the kind of healing I needed to do. I could be alone but not feel alone.

With the condo squared away as a temporary housing solution, there was still the issue of the van buildout. Even if I didn't end up living in it full time, I wanted to have a few creature comforts installed for future camping trips.

While the timing wasn't optimal, I managed to get a build slot for the first phase of the van conversion the day after Labor Day—the same day I moved into the condo. That would leave me without transportation until the buildout was complete, which meant I'd have to rely on the beach trolley and Uber in the interim.

But I'd have to postpone celebrating the condo, and the fact that my life was starting to come together. In just a couple more days, I'd be on a flight to Seattle to finalize my divorce.

In some ways, the days leading up to my divorce felt like they'd flown by, but in other ways it felt like it had taken years. So much had happened since I rolled down my driveway on the day of closing. And it was hard to believe that was already more than two months ago.

My flight back to Seattle gave me some time to think about a lot of things. A change of scenery always has a way of putting things into perspective for me. Breaking out of my familiar routines and environments has always helped me think more clearly. It's one of the reasons I bought van.

My mind drifted back to Byron Katie's teachings in her book *Loving What Is*. No matter how I felt about my marriage ending, it *was* going to end. Even so, I was anxious to get the documents signed so I could go on with my life.

At the airport, I picked up my rental car and headed toward Salish Lodge & Spa, a chic boutique hotel overlooking Snoqualmie Falls.

The hotel wasn't far from my old home in Issaquah. When I lived there, I visited the spa frequently. Aside from the luxurious spa treatments, I equally loved relaxing in the indoor, heated saltwater pool. It made the cold, rainy days more bearable. But with the proximity being so close to home, I'd never had a reason to stay at the lodge. It somehow felt appropriate now, on the night before I'd stand next to my husband one last time, to splurge and book a room there.

Before settling into my room, I took a short walk down to the falls, hoping the misty air would somehow help me clear my head. I stood behind the railing of the overlook, and watched the water pour down over the rocky edge, softly at first, and then gaining momentum as it rushed over the edge of the cliff. I recognized that rush. The intensity felt familiar. I'd recently jumped headfirst into my own pool of chaos. But I was slowly drifting downstream, to where the water was much calmer.

I meandered down the path that led back to the hotel, snapping pictures of summer flowers along the way. I loved the summer months in Washington. Nature exploded into bursts of color that somehow made the dark winter days worth it.

I made my way back to the hotel and wandered into the dining room, where I placed a to-go order. For some reason, I felt like spending the evening alone, without the laughter of tourists distracting me from my sadness. While I waited, I sipped on a glass of wine while I looked out the window over the falls.

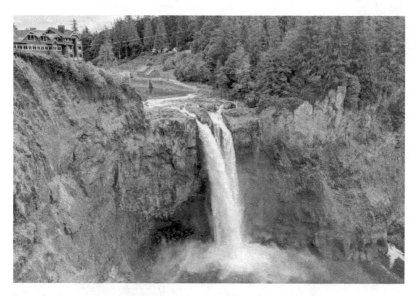

*Overlooking Salish Falls in Snoqualmie, WA*

When I returned to my room, I wrapped myself in the fuzzy robe I found hanging in the closet. It wasn't quite as comforting and familiar as my own robe, but it would have to do. I turned on the electric fireplace before curling up in the leather chair beside the bed. I poured myself another glass of wine, and then poured my heart out onto the pages of my journal.

*How and why in the actual fuck am I sitting alone in this hotel room right now? How did we let this happen?*

As I sobbed my final tears as a married woman, it felt good to release the resurgence of emotions. Being surrounded by old memories made it hard to forget that I'd be letting go of them completely in the morning.

In less than 24 hours, I'd be reclaiming my maiden name—for the second time in my adult life. But it felt good. I'd never quite understood why I decided to hyphenate my name when I got married the second time anyway, but maybe it was an early sign that I wasn't fully invested in the relationship. Maybe my first failed marriage had left more scars than I realized.

I wrote a goodbye letter to my soon-to-be ex-husband, hoping that it would somehow help me sort through some of the lingering hurt that wouldn't quite budge. I scrawled out a few lines in my journal, but when I stared back at the words on the pages, they felt gross. They were full of anger and blame and judgement.

I tossed the letter into the trash can near the coffee pot and started a letter to my future self instead. Onto a blank page I spilled words of encouragement and strength and hope. I reminded myself how far I had come in such a short time and how important these lessons would be for my growth. I reminded myself that every moment—whether or not I could see the good in them yet—was a gift. Each moment was leading me closer to my highest good.

When the words no longer flowed easily, I climbed into the soft sheets of the hotel bed next to me. If acceptance had a feeling, I imagined that's what it felt like. Cozy, warm, and peaceful.

It was only 3 a.m. when I opened my eyes. The time change always threw me for a loop. It was still dark outside, but I was wide awake. I walked over to the coffee station and made a pour-over, and then grabbed my journal from the bedside table.

Feeling hungry, I took a shower and headed to the dining room, where I had a lovely breakfast overlooking the falls. Afterward, I returned to my room and did a brief grounding meditation before I gathered my things and headed down to pick up the rental car from the valet.

# Divorced

I felt calm and ready. But the moment I sat down behind the wheel of the rental car, I instantly felt nauseous. I thought I was ready to tug on the last string to complete our unraveling, but I felt more waves of sadness creep in. I took a few deep breaths and flashed a fake smile at the valet attendant, who had been watching me from the curbside. I put the car into gear and turned toward the highway.

When I arrived at the courthouse parking garage, I pulled into an empty space and removed the keys from the ignition. I arrived early on purpose, expecting that I'd need some extra time to gather my composure. I took a few more deep breaths and quietly savored the last few moments of calm before I'd have to face my husband one last time.

I closed my eyes and imagined my life just a few short months before. I imagined myself out running a few simple errands, returning to my beautiful home, and being greeted by my cute miniature dachshund, who would have been waiting for me with her tail wagging wildly. I missed Zoey. In fact, I realized that I hadn't yet grieved her passing. There were too many other chaotic pieces of my life to put back into place.

In the six years that I'd lived in Washington State, I'd had my share of both beautiful and heartbreaking experiences. But this one today felt surreal.

As I opened my eyes, I reminded myself that while our marriage was about to come to an end legally, it had been over long before I pulled into that parking garage. It had been on life support for years. We'd only pretended it was still alive, propping it up like a character in *Weekend at Bernie's*, hoping things would somehow get better on their own. But hoping hadn't helped. Things hadn't gotten better. And in just a few more minutes, our divorce would be final, leaving us both free to explore the next chapters of our lives separately.

And then I thought back to a realization I'd made earlier, just after we made the decision to uncouple: What brought me joy, brought *him* suffering. And what brought him joy, brought *me* suffering. That was the reality we'd been unwilling or unable to acknowledge.

But we'd both suffered enough.

I sat clutching the keys and watching the hands on my watch tick closer to the point when I'd be forced to open the door and start walking. It had been three months since I'd watched from the living room window as his taillights disappeared at the end of the driveway.

In truth, I wasn't even sure if he would be there. The court only required one of us to be present in person. Early on, he'd said that he planned to be there, but in the back of my mind, I worried that if something came up and he couldn't make it, the date would only get pushed back further. I wasn't willing to risk that. I needed closure, and delaying the inevitable was pointless.

But I also wasn't sure how I'd react if he did show up. Would I break down in tears? Would I feel angry? Would I feel heartbroken? I pulled the keys from the ignition and began walking toward the front steps of the courthouse. Once inside, I stepped through the security line x-ray machine and then took the elevator upstairs to the pre-assigned room.

I was early, so I found a seat on a bench just outside the door in the hallway. A couple of minutes later my phone dinged and a text message appeared.

It was him.

"Are you here?" it said.

I hadn't told him I was coming. In fact, we hadn't spoken in months. We'd only exchanged a few transactional messages.

But before I could respond to the text, my phone rang, and I reluctantly answered it.

He was on his way up.

My heart raced. I wished he hadn't come.

When I looked up from my phone a couple minutes later, I saw him slowly walking toward me from the other end of the hallway. It was odd to look into the eyes of a man that I was still married to and feel nothing at all. But that's how I felt. When he was finally standing in front of me, I felt absolutely nothing. No anger. No endearment. Only indifference.

In fact, I barely recognized him. Nothing about him seemed familiar. He could have just as easily been a stranger I'd never seen before. I felt relieved. I'd been prepared to feel something. But I certainly hadn't expected to feel nothing.

After a few random pleasantries, we opened the door to the courtroom and found some seats near the aisle. The room was filled with strangers who, like us, were waiting for their turn to stand before the judge.

When the judge finally called our names, I felt queasy again. I swallowed hard as we both stood and made our way toward the raised wooden desk at the front of the room. I felt like a criminal standing there beside a man I didn't know.

After confirming our names and the details of our case, the judge asked us to verbalize our agreement that the marriage was, indeed, irretrievably broken.

*Irretrievably broken.*

I'd never thought of it that way. But it was, indeed, irretrievable.

Then, with a quick stroke of a pen and a couple stamps of ink, our lives were forever changed. The judge then handed off the documents to a court staff member, and called out the name of the next case in line.

That was it.

In less than two minutes, we'd gone from being a married couple to two strangers who would likely never see each other again. The high school flame that we'd so hopefully reignited was now fully extinguished. And we were free to go on with our lives.

Together, we walked to the clerk's office to pick up copies of our official divorce decree. When the clerk handed me my copy, I stared down at my maiden name on the paper.

It was a relief to finally have that chapter of my life closed, and I was grateful that I hadn't experienced the emotional meltdown I'd prepared myself for. In the weeks leading up to the court date, I had carefully planned a series of post-divorce self-care strategies. I think that helped.

My first stop after the courthouse was at a cold-pressed juice bar in Issaquah, where I enjoyed some lovely lavender almond milk and spent a few minutes debriefing in my journal. Afterward, I made my way back to my friend's retreat center, where Janene would be arriving later to give me another 2-hour massage, just as she had six weeks before.

I'd learned over the past several years of honing my self-care practice that having something to look forward to was critical, especially when my emotions were raw and fragile.

At the end of the day, and after my luxurious massage, I felt peaceful. I felt grounded. And even though the divorce created yet another loss, I felt whole.

The next morning, I realized that I was finally excited about my future, a feeling that I hadn't felt since picking up the van at the dealership.

# Maiden

I was first in line when the license bureau opened the following day. In my hands I gripped a manila file folder that held proof of my name change—no more hyphen.

I liked seeing my maiden name displayed across my driver's license, but I wasn't looking forward to the work ahead of me.

Having already been through one divorce, I remembered just how time consuming and grueling it was. I wasn't looking forward to it. Every time I felt certain that I'd updated the last of my accounts, I'd find one more that needed to be updated. Everything—my mailing address, account numbers, checks, licenses, titles, beneficiaries—all of it would have to be changed.

And because I still wasn't sure if I would stay in Florida after my lease was up at the condo, I decided to keep my mailbox address in Washington State. For all I knew, I'd be making a return trip after my extended vacation was over. I still wasn't ready to make any big decisions about a permanent home yet.

Later, I met up with a group of friends for an early dinner, and then returned to my hotel, which was located near the airport. I had an early flight the next morning, so I repacked most of my things before bed to make things easier.

In the morning, I dropped off the rental car at the airport and grabbed some breakfast and coffee before taking a seat at my gate. I arrived about an hour early to avoid feeling rushed. I hadn't realized how much I detested rushing to the gate for so many years of my married life.

But something had shifted overnight. Maybe it was the 2-hour massage, and maybe it was simply that the divorce was now final. But whatever it was, I felt a sense of ease. My spirit felt happy to finally be untethered. I was free.

By the time my flight arrived back in Tampa, I felt stronger. I felt more like myself. And I had everything I needed to start over again.

I had officially reclaimed my independence—and my name—back in Seattle, but the acceptance piece was proving to be more challenging than I imagined. I wrongly assumed that once the papers were signed and the ink was dry that I'd somehow no longer feel sadness. But it lingered.

Some days I struggled more than others. It seemed like each time I made progress with designing my future, a memory from the past would bull-doze me over.

Those were the moments when I realized that I missed the man I married, but not the man I left. It was true. The man I left was not the man I fell in love with when I was seventeen, nor was he the man I fell in love with again in my late twenties.

I suspected that he felt the same way about me. In our twelve years together, we'd grown apart in so many different ways.

What I missed the most wasn't the marriage itself. It was more than that. What I missed the most was the life I'd build over the course of our marriage. I'd spent so many years of my life building friendships, building a business, and building a life. I'd lost more than just a partner; I'd lost a community. And I'd also lost my identity.

# North Carolina

Since I had some time before moving into the condo, I decided to make a quick trip to Ohio to visit my dad. Living on the West Coast for so many years had made it difficult to visit family members who lived on the other side of the country. Now that I was closer, I thought it made sense to make up for some lost time.

Before leaving Issaquah, I joined an RV membership community called Harvest Hosts. Members are able to camp for free at wineries, breweries, distilleries, farms, and museums throughout the country. And while there are no camping fees per se, you're expected to support the host in some way, whether it's through volunteering or purchasing something at the winery.

I hadn't yet found a host location along my route from Seattle, but there were several prospects between Florida and Ohio. Excited to try it out, I reserved my first stay at Grove Winery in Gibsonville, NC.

I pulled into the parking area near the tasting room and quickly found a spot at the end of the lot. I carefully positioned the van so that I had a beautiful view of the vineyard when the door was open.

The tasting room was small, and there were already two other couples sitting at the bar, so I ordered a glass of Nebbiolo and wandered outside to find a place to sit in the sun. In the distance, there was an outdoor stage next to a small pond. I'd read on the website that on weekends they held live outdoor music events. Since it was a weekday, it was much quieter.

I found an open metal table that had been warming in the sun and sat down to enjoy the view. North Carolina was still on my list of potential places to relocate, despite my earlier mishap at the campground a few weeks prior. I was looking at the Raleigh area, which was a little over an hour east of the winery. I loved the idea of being able to spend time in the mountains or near the ocean, depending on my mood. It reminded me of Seattle.

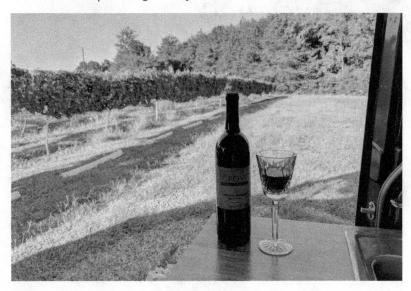

*Stacy's campsite at Grove Winery in Gibsonville, NC*

When my glass was empty, I returned to the tasting room to purchase a bottle of Nebbiolo for later. After I placed my order, a woman who was sitting at the bar had overheard that I was camping in my van overnight.

"I love that you're doing that," she said.

"Yeah, it's been interesting," I said. I relayed that I'd made my way across the country, along with a few of the highlights of my trip.

"You know, women are far more capable than a lot of people give us credit for," she said. "I drove an 18-wheeler for several years and that was quite the experience."

She looked nothing like what I imagined an 18-wheeler-driving woman would look like, but then again, I'd never met one before now.

I ordered another glass of wine and we shared stories of our adventures on the road. We'd both agreed that just about anything is possible if you want it badly enough. The only limits we run into are the ones we set in our own minds. Life is unlimited. The conversation was the boost I needed, offering me hope that the trip would eventually lead me wherever I needed to be.

I returned to the van to prepare some pasta to go with my wine. I'd recently ordered a new Jetboil Minimo camp stove that I was excited to try out for the first time. The two burner Coleman stove that I'd been using was much bigger, and it required me to set up a table outside. Most of the time that was fine, unless the weather wasn't great, or I just didn't feel like doing it. The Jetboil is ultra fast—boiling water in about a minute—making it much easier to make coffee and tea as well.

After dinner, I prepared my bed for the night and curled up in my sleeping bag. Up to that point, my favorite places to camp had been state parks, but Harvest Hosts venues were already becoming a close second. While the winery didn't offer any amenities, like bathrooms or showers, I felt safe there. And that made all the difference.

# Ohio

My visit to Ohio was short but sweet. It was great to reconnect with friends and family that I hadn't seen since my life was turned upside down. Some had been concerned about my well-being, and having a chance to sit down and share some of my travel stories with them did us both some good.

But in the back of my mind, I couldn't wait to get back to Florida. I was eager to lay down some temporary roots in the condo and spend some time sorting out my options from the balcony.

On my way back to Florida, I decided to make a quick stop to see a friend in Kentucky and then venture down to Chattanooga, a city I'd never had a chance to visit before. There, I drove up to Lookout Mountain for a picturesque view of the city, and returned to the main highway for the last leg. I had something to look forward to again and I was anxious to get back.

Since I'd be dropping off the van with the builder the same day I moved into the condo, I had to completely unload everything. And that meant my mom's garage would have to serve as a temporary storage unit until the van was done. Although I'd downsized quite a bit already, the unloading process was just as unpleasant as the loading process had been back in Issaquah.

My life had become a constant juggle, and I felt unsettled. Thankfully, the condo was completely furnished, so I'd only need to bring clothes, food, and a few personal items. It was simple. And I'd grown to adore simple.

# The Condo

After dropping off the van in Deland, FL, my mom and I made our way down to Clearwater Beach to get me moved into the condo.

The view from the top of the bridge on the way to the beach was beautiful. The blue-green water shimmered in the sunlight while the palm trees swayed gently on both sides of the highway. Two bridges are all that connect the mainland to the beach, so technically it's an island. And I was all sorts of ready for a transition to island life.

As we drove, high school memories came flooding back: cruising on the beach in my Honda Accord and hating the fact that I had a curfew, my best friend accidently spraying me in the face with pepper spray while testing out the new safety device on her keychain, and a few sunset kisses on the beach with high school crushes. It was hard to imagine myself at 17 again. That was 25 years ago.

We arrived at the condo and it took no time at all to put away the few items I'd brought along. Aside from my clothes, I brought my laptop, so I could continue my work at LivingUpp; a handful of journals that I had little doubt I'd fill quickly; my French press; a yoga mat; a pair of binoculars for dolphin and bird watching; an afghan for warmth and comfort; a few books; and a little black dress—just in case. You never know.

I didn't need anything else. The condo was completely furnished, and the kitchen was fully stocked, with the exception of food and wine. I was all set for four months.

I figured that if I discovered something was missing, I could always grab a few more items at my mom's house when I returned to pick up the van.

After saying goodbye to my mom, I found a wine glass in the kitchen and poured some Riesling into it. Then I made my way out to the balcony. I couldn't wait to soak in the calming energy of the ocean and the warmth of the sun.

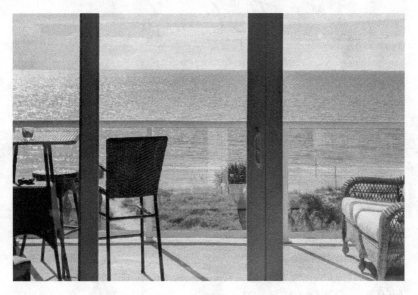

*A view from the condo balcony*

Outside on the balcony, there were several seating options: a cushioned wicker couch, two cushioned wicker chairs, and a high-top table with four wicker stools. I climbed up onto one of the stools and stretched out my legs on another one in front of me. They both felt warm from the afternoon sun. I glanced down at my phone and saw that it was 91 degrees.

Florida temperatures in early September far exceed Seattle's mid-summer temperatures. Like, by a lot. On my weather app, I punched in Issaquah just to see what the temperature was there. My eyes widened when I saw that the projected high was 68. The overnight low at the beach wouldn't even fall below 75.

I took another sip from my wine glass, which was now completely covered in condensation from the warm air, and closed my eyes, relishing my new reality for the next four months.

The previous five months had been filled with adrenaline-fueled anxiety, and the stress had been building up within me. While I had a few healthy outlets for the negative energy through various forms of self-care, like massage, journaling, and physical activity, the healing that I still needed to do would require a much bigger investment.

My trip had given me the space to begin accepting my new reality. Now, I was finally ready to release my role as the victim, and begin the real work of forgiveness.

Soon, the ocean's salty, humid air stirred memories and emotions within me. I recalled sitting on the cold rocks on Ruby Beach just two months earlier, and how I felt looking out at the cold ocean. Now, staring out at a much warmer ocean, it mirrored back the warmth I was finally beginning to feel again.

On the road, I had been free to express my emotions. After driving all day, I looked forward to the evening release. A good cry always made me feel better. But I didn't feel comfortable crying in front of other people, so staying with family for the past six weeks had left few opportunities for the tears to flow.

But there was nothing holding back the tears now. I could tell that crying and drinking wine on the balcony would soon become an afternoon ritual. There, I felt safe to sift through the uncomfortable memories, doing my best to make sense of everything that had happened.

It offered a slow release valve for the layers of sadness that had accumulated within me, and it gave me a safe place to move through the uncomfortable memories that I had allowed to steal my joy for far too long. I hoped to be able to untangle everything, to at least make some sense of it, and to extract the lessons that I needed to move forward.

I thought about all of the soul-searching and personal growth I'd invested in over the past few years, trying to find the answer to the looming question: *Should I stay, or should I go?*

In my quest for answers, I turned to God, to my therapist, to family and friends, to *A Course in Miracles*, and to meditation. I'd even met with a Shamanic healer in hopes of making sense of the mess that my life had become.

I was struggling with how to handle my unhappiness, but I hadn't realized I was seeking answers to questions that I still wasn't ready to answer. Looking back, perhaps all of it was helping to prepare me for the unavoidable transition that led me here.

# The Ocean Fixes Everything

A couple days after moving into the condo, I noticed a little block of wood on the bathroom counter with the words *The Ocean Fixes Everything* painted on the front of it. It made me smile. In the two days that I'd been there I hadn't noticed it. The ocean really was fixing me. I could feel it.

Being at the condo meant that I no longer had to find a new place to stay every night, and that was a relief. I hadn't realized how much anxiety I'd been experiencing on the road. Planting some roots, even if just temporarily, felt really good. Shallow roots were better than none at all. I'd enjoyed my time on the road, but it was nice to feel grounded again. I was ready to relax and give my body a chance to recover. The ocean was exactly what I needed.

The sound of the waves offered me peace. But I was still numb inside. I still needed to process everything that had happened, but I was getting impatient with myself.

I just wanted to feel good again. The heaviness of feeling not good enough, not attractive enough, and not important enough to fight for, weighed heavily on my soul. I had doubts that I'd ever feel joyful again.

The days that included afternoon thundershowers were my favorite. I'd sit on the balcony and feel the mist from the rain surround me. The cooler air felt chilly for a brief moment before returning to the sweltering humidity from before.

And the warmth. I relished the warmth. I started to see that the coldness of the life I'd left behind was about more than just the temperature; it was about how I felt.

I spent a lot of time reflecting on how everything had unfolded in such a short amount of time. I recalled each momentous milestone that had gotten me here—our decision to uncouple, the sale of our home, the loss of our beloved Zoey, my decision to buy the van and take a spontaneous trip across the country, and the manifestation of the condo I would be living in for the next few weeks.

All of it had happened in just five short months.

In those twenty weeks, my life had gone from safe and secure to upended and open ended. I hadn't realized how much heaviness I was still carrying. Some of the memories were still painfully tender and would no doubt take time to sort through.

As part of my morning practice, I continued to study *A Course in Miracles*. It slowly helped me reframe the events and choices that had been made, a process that I now refer to as reflect-release-realign. And in that process, I began to slowly recover my sense of myself.

My days consisted of walks on the beach, yoga, meditation, preparing nourishing meals, journaling, staying in touch with friends, and helping other women build a solid self-care foundation through my work at LivingUpp.

When I looked at myself in the mirror, I saw a calm, grounded woman who had everything she needed. Now I just needed to figure out exactly what I wanted my life to be like—what I wanted to do, be, have, and feel.

I had no doubts that my strong foundation of self-care was going to help me figure it out.

# Red Tide

While the van was with the builder, I relied on the Jolley Trolley, a local beach shuttle that looped up and down the beach all day. Once a week or so, I'd hop on the trolley to get a few groceries. It wasn't optimal, but I'd grown used to figuring out how to deal with less than optimal conditions. By that point, I was confident that I could find a solution for just about anything.

My first week at the beach had been blissful, but by the second week, red tide had progressively gotten worse in the area. Each morning when I opened the sliding glass door, the overpowering scent of dead fish and putrid air wafted in. It blanketed the beach. There was no escaping it.

From my balcony, I could see shimmering objects bobbing on the water's surface. They were dead fish slowly making their way to shore. Beach crews worked relentlessly on a daily basis to clean up the shoreline. From morning to night, beachcombers rolled up and down the beach, scooping up everything the waves tossed onto the sand.

Despite the foulness of it all, I'd learned how to go with the flow. I laughed to myself about the odds of there being a red tide during my short stay at the condo. Even so, the view from the balcony was still amazing, and I was determined to make the most of my time there.

Morning walks on the beach became part of my morning self-care practice. I'd wake up around 5 a.m., press a pot of coffee and have a cup or two on the balcony before taking the elevator downstairs to the beach.

I loved being an early riser. On most days, I made it down to the sand before the sun was out. After my hour-long walk, I'd return to the balcony to watch shell hunters, joggers, and beachcombers make their way up and down the beach.

Walking along the shoreline reminded me that everything meaningful happens on the edge—edges of the forest, edges of town, edges of the ocean. Edges are where endings and beginnings meet, like so many of life's meaningful transitions.

Recently, I'd been forced to walk on a lot of edges, but I knew that it was all for my highest good.

During my walks on the beach, I watched blue herons and snowy egrets. I saw dolphins emerge from the water in the distance. And I felt the fine, powdery sand between my toes. On a daily basis, it always led me back to one truth: It's really hard to be sad at the beach.

Since the worsening red tide kept me from spending as much time outside as I would have liked, I decided to develop my first online course. The 8-week self-care program was a collection of everything I'd learned throughout my personal self-care journey, and now I'd get to teach other women how to weave elements of self-care into their own lives. I saw just how important and powerful it was to have grounding daily self-care rituals during life's big transitions.

The time inside also gave me more time to journal. Seeing my thoughts on paper helped me assess them for truth. I felt frustrated that I didn't yet have a clear vision of what to do when I left the condo.

My heart seemed to know what it needed: more time.

But patience hasn't always been my greatest virtue. The truth is, all of my *doing* over the years had interfered with my *being*. My constant busyness kept me from enjoying and celebrating the beautiful moments and milestones of my life. I was starting to learn that now. I no longer wanted to waste the precious moments of my life lamenting the past or fretting about the future.

I was just beginning to learn the art of suffering, but I wondered how much longer the suffering was going to last. I was tired of feeling sad. I was tired of grieving.

As I began to dive deeper into the lessons that were wrapped up in the end of my marriage, I experienced a wide range of emotions. Anger came in waves. I was angry that the fairy tale marriage I'd created in my mind hadn't played out that way. I was angry that I was forced to completely redesign my life, while the only thing he had to change was his address.

And I felt sad. I felt sad that he hadn't fought harder to keep me—although I wasn't exactly sure what that might have looked like. I mean, he'd done everything I'd asked of him. He'd read books that we'd later discussed together. He attended therapy sessions. He'd done the things he said he was willing to do.

But the question was, had *I*? Yes, outwardly I'd done all of those same things, but inside I hadn't forgiven him. And I certainly didn't trust him. Without those two vital pieces, it seemed unrealistic to think that a foundation could be rebuilt in any relationship, let alone a marriage.

The truth was, I hadn't invested as much in the marriage as I wanted to believe I had.

And I also knew that holding onto the anger and bitterness and sadness wasn't going to serve anyone. I needed to release the negative charge I still carried.

For years, I'd gone to great lengths to avoid the elephant in the room: that I had also played a role in the affair. While I was in no way responsible for anyone's actions or choices other than my own, I most certainly shared responsibility for creating the conditions that led to the erosion of our relationship. And unless I was willing to own that, then I couldn't change my experience of my reality.

I also couldn't ignore the reality that the reason I'd felt so unloved for so long, was that I wasn't able to receive what I wasn't able to give in the first place. Love attracts love.

Yes, I'd been betrayed. But so had he. I hadn't shown up as the person that I vowed to be in the marriage, either. The truth that I'd been unwilling to face was that I betrayed him, too.

Even so, I knew deep down that the biggest betrayal of all was my betrayal of myself. I'd betrayed myself by staying silent when I knew early on that something was wrong. My intuition had sensed it, and yet I'd chosen to ignore it. I'd convinced myself that it was just one of the many phases a relationship goes through, the ever-evolving cycle of connection and disconnection. And instead of openly discussing it, I'd suppressed my feelings to the point that I felt bitter and angry most of the time.

I'd betrayed myself to the point that I could no longer trust my own judgement, let alone anyone else's. It was becoming clear to me that everything I thought he'd done to me, I'd also done to myself.

I'd betrayed myself in my unwillingness to admit earlier in the relationship that I was unhappy. I'd been unwilling to have the uncomfortable conversation to address my unhappiness. I'd even been unwilling to see that he had feelings for someone else, until it was too late. Instead of using my voice, I'd pretended nothing was wrong.

And that's where self-care came in. I journaled. I walked on the beach. I meditated. I practiced yoga. I tended to each of the 8 dimensions of my life. And little by little, I released the identity of the betrayed victim that I'd been clinging to for the past few years.

While sitting on the balcony one afternoon, I received an email saying the van was ready for pickup. I called my mom and coordinated a return trip to Deland to pick up the van. I honestly don't know what I would have done without the help of my family.

A few days later, we arrived at the builder's shop and the van was already outside charging.

It looked like a brand-new van. It had flooring, walls, ceiling fans, an awning, and a 12-volt electrical system that would allow me to install a fridge and charge my devices from the road. It was starting to look like an actual tiny home.

When I returned to my mother's house, we loaded up the van with a few more of my things before heading back to the beach. I felt a renewed sense of excitement—not just about designing the interior of the van, but about designing my life.

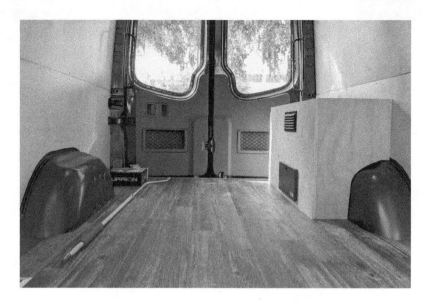

*Phase I of the van buildout*

# A Cold Bed

Another friend flew in for a short weekend visit. Jaime and I had known each other since junior high, and she was one of the few childhood friends I'd managed to stay connected with in my adult life.

One evening during her visit, we'd planned to have an early dinner at a local restaurant, and then wander back down the beach for some sunset cocktails on the balcony at the condo.

I hadn't worn a dress since my trip to Paris back in January, and I felt ready to wear something other than yoga pants. I put on the one black dress that I'd taken with me to the condo, and slid on a pair of heels. I curled my hair. I put on jewelry. And for the first time since all hell had broken loose, I felt good.

We took the Jolley Trolley down to the beach, made our way to the host stand at the restaurant, and then found a seat at the bar to have a cocktail before dinner.

Not long after we sat down, a white-haired, older man took a seat at the far end of the bar. It was clear that the bartender knew him since he promptly brought him a drink without taking his order.

"Are you all from here?" he asked.

Jaime shared that she was visiting from Ohio, and then he turned and looked at me.

"I'm a gypsy," I said. I'd learned that simply saying I was a nomad who was just passing through was easier than telling the whole truth about why I was renting a condo on the beach.

"A gypsy?" he asked.

"Well, I just got divorced and thought some time at the beach might do me some good," I said.

He raised his eyebrows a little and said, "You know," he paused, which I was certain he did to ensure he'd gotten my full attention. "A man doesn't leave a warm bed for a cold one."

The corners of his mouth curled upward a little, clearly satisfied with his assessment of me. He picked up the glass in front of him, which held an amber-colored liquid, and then took a sip before returning it to the bar.

"Neither does a woman," I said, staring directly back at him.

His head had been tilted down toward his glass, but his eyes moved up to meet mine. I was glad we got that squared away.

After dinner, Jaime and I kicked off our heels and headed toward the beach. We'd decided to walk back to the condo rather than taking the trolley. The beach is lovely just before sunset.

The next day, weather reports issued a warning of a hurricane approaching the Gulf. And because conditions continued to worsen, Jaime decided to book an earlier flight home to avoid travel delays.

Just like the red tide, I hadn't factored a hurricane into my time at the beach. In fact, I'd already made plans for the weekend. On what would have been my 8th wedding anniversary, I'd planned to sit alone on the pier drinking a bottle of Veuve Clicquot to celebrate my independence.

I hated to leave the beach, but it seemed like the sensible thing to do. My mom's house was further inland, and since the van is so high-profile, the wind could be damaging even without threats of high water.

Plus, I already had plans to head back to Ohio the following weekend to begin the next phase of the van buildout with my dad's help. Leaving a day or two earlier wasn't going to make that much difference. I brought the balcony furniture inside the condo and secured it in the living room, and then locked the sliding glass door behind me before heading north to my mom's.

# A Black Eye

After the threat of the storm had passed, I booked an overnight stay at a small Harvest Hosts site near the halfway point on my trip to Ohio. The Carolina Heritage Vineyard & Winery located in Elkin, NC holds the title of being the first certified organic winery in North Carolina.

I happened to arrive in the middle of harvest season, which meant I got to help pick grapes at the vineyard alongside the owners and their crew.

Pat and Clyde were delightful tour guides, and it was fascinating to see how much work goes into being a vintner. After Pat guided me through a wine flight in the tasting room and I selected a bottle to enjoy later that evening, I returned to the van to rest up for the final leg of my trip to Ohio.

I drifted off to sleep envisioning what the van would look like when it was finished: my very own writing cottage on wheels.

For Ohio, it was unseasonably cold that early in the season, with temperatures dipping down into the 30s overnight. And with regards to the van buildout, that presented a few extra challenges, particularly because cold hands don't maneuver well.

For three days, we measured and cut boards, and cussed when we discovered we needed to recut boards. He had the tools, and I had the vision.

It became evident soon after my dad and I began the project that we weren't the most ideal project team. Neither of us are the most patient souls, and we'd later confess that we both felt rushed by the other. Nevertheless, we got the job done—but not without a few injuries.

In addition to the cold weather, my limited experience using power tools, coupled with my dad's overestimation of my abilities, landed him with a black eye and a smallish arm wound. Buy in the end, the finished product was perfect.

First, we built a platform, so I had plenty of room to store gear beneath it. In a lot of the DIY van builds I'd seen, there seemed to be a lot of wasted space, and I wanted to have room to store clothing, food, cooking equipment, cleaning supplies, and tools.

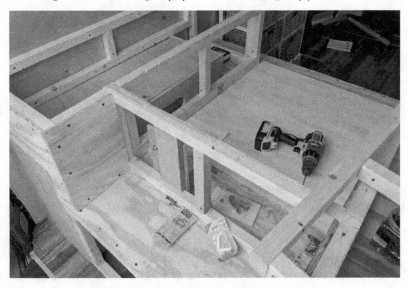

*Phase II of the van buildout*

On top of the platform, we built a u-shaped bench seat that can be converted into a bed at night, and each of the bench tops were hinged to allow for storage inside. I wanted to be able to store my sheets, blankets, and pillows where I could access them easily. Inside the middle of the "u," we installed a Lagun swivel table, which can be lowered to become part of the bed platform.

The project was intense, but we were both still alive at the end of it. And I was beyond thrilled with the finished product. It was exactly what I'd hoped for. With the foundation for the bed, table, and storage in place, the rest of the buildout was mostly decorative. All that was left was installing a heater and adding some cushions for the bedding.

When it was time to head back to Florida, I loaded up the van and said my goodbyes. I was excited to spend my first night stretched out on the new bed platform instead of the cold floor. I set my map to Pine Level, NC, where I planned to spend the night at another Harvest Hosts winery.

After a lovely glass of Muscadine wine in the Hinnant Farms Vineyard & Winery tasting room, and another bottle to go, I walked back to the van to settle in for the night. Weather reports were still predicting cold temperatures overnight, and I was still without a source of heat unless the van was running, so getting to bed early was my only hope to stay warm.

I laid out my sleeping pad on the new wooden platform, and then layered my sleeping bag and blankets on top. I wasn't sure what I was expecting, but it really wasn't any more comfortable than the floor had been. It definitely needed cushions. But at least I didn't have to lie directly on top of the chilly rubber mat anymore.

As I shivered myself to sleep, my thoughts drifted back to the Florida condo, and the warm, salty air on the balcony. I missed the beach. I'd grown used to hearing the sound of the ocean, and feeling the warmth of the sun.

# Luxurious

When I got back to the condo, I was relieved that a few more pieces of my life seemed to be falling into place. With the van buildout almost complete, all that was left was figuring out where to go when I left the condo.

But as I approached my third month there, I couldn't help but feel a twinge of fear. Three months had flown by, and with just a month left at the condo, I still hadn't decided where to go next. I'd been looking seriously at Raleigh, NC since before leaving Seattle, but I wasn't sure that I really wanted to move to a city where I knew absolutely no one. Plus, I also couldn't shake the unpleasant feelings I still had about being disturbed in the middle of the night while camping not far from there.

The van gave me options, but it didn't give me answers. It had only been a temporary solution to buy me more time. But my time was running out.

I made arrangements to have my mom help me with the third phase of the van buildout, which involved sewing the cushions and curtains. I wanted to make the van feel cozy. Sleeping on pieces of rough plywood wasn't exactly the luxury experience I'd envisioned.

While I never planned on being a full-time van dweller, it eased my mind just knowing that I had a safe place to sleep if I ever needed one. And even if I only ended up taking periodic weekend trips, comfort was non-negotiable. I'd roughed it long enough.

After measuring at least a dozen times, I purchased the pre-cut foam for the cushions at a local upholstery shop, and then picked up some fabric. One fabric was a black and cream buffalo check pattern, and the other was a travel themed pattern, with the names of cities from all around the globe printed on it. I planned to use the fabric for the curtains, pillows, and cushions.

I'd already scored a plush rug at HomeGoods that fit perfectly inside the u-shaped area, and after putting it in place, I stood back to marvel at the transformation. It didn't even look like the same van I'd traveled across the country in.

I felt tearful, seeing what I'd envisioned for months now manifested right in front of me. It felt like home. And it felt luxurious.

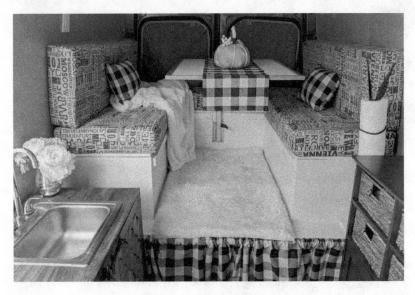

*Phase III of the van buildout*

When I returned to the condo, I poured myself a glass of Riesling and headed straight to the balcony. I doubted that I could ever tire of the beautiful ocean view.

Tears came without warning. Except this time, they weren't sad tears. They were joyful tears. My life finally felt like it was coming together. I was relieved to have the van buildout mostly complete, and I still had some time left at the condo to plan my next adventure.

# Manatees

A few days later, another friend flew in for a weekend getaway. Tawnya and I met in college, where we worked together as banquet servers at Kent State University. Her extreme extroverted nature couldn't be more opposite from mine, but we always had fun whenever we got together.

One of the activities we'd planned for the weekend was to go swimming with manatees, something that had been on my bucket list since I was a kid. In the winter months, manatees flock to Crystal River near Homosassa Springs, where the water is warmer, staying at close to 72 degrees year-round.

By Florida standards it was cold, which meant we'd probably start the morning wearing long sleeves and then be comfortable in bathing suits by the time the sun peeked above the horizon. It was my kind of cold.

With the chilly ambient temperatures, it also meant that the water would feel slightly warmer, comparatively speaking. But for a chance to see manatees close-up, I was willing to be chilly.

We boarded the charter boat and made our way to the area of the river where manatees frequently congregated. After gearing up with our snorkeling masks and water shoes, we hoisted ourselves over the side of the boat and plunged into the cold water. It was colder than I expected, but I adjusted quickly.

The water was murky—so murky that it was difficult to see more than a couple feet in front of us. Each time a manatee came into view, it was a complete shock. One minute I was floating quietly in a sea of algae, and the next an oddly shaped muzzle would appear in front of my face. To say that I squealed like a six-year-old would be putting it mildly. My heart raced and my breath quickened, and I smiled like an idiot beneath the water's surface.

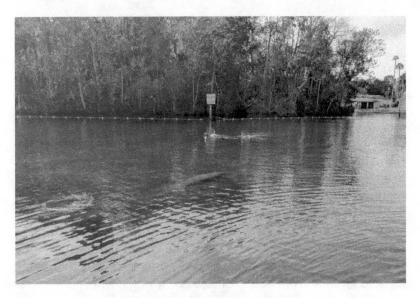

*Snorkeling with manatees at Homosassa Springs, FL*

After several close encounters, we made our way back to the boat, where we watched from above as more manatees continued to swirl around us. Thankfully, it didn't take long for the sun to warm our bodies on the deck.

When we returned to the condo, we had some cocktails on the balcony while we planned out the rest of our evening.

"Do you have any desire at all to start dating again?" Tawnya asked.

I almost spit out my wine.

"Um, no," I said quickly. I didn't even need to think about it. I wasn't interested at all in being in a relationship again. Part of me thought I never would be.

All of my friends were curious about the same thing, but I

wasn't interested in anything that threatened my newfound independence. I'd grown quite fond of not needing to notify anyone of my whereabouts, ask for input on the color of my van interior, or agree on what to have for dinner.

I'd been adjusting to life as a single woman just fine. In fact, the mere sight of couples holding hands on the beach made me want to vomit. I'd see their smiling, naive faces and wonder if they had any idea what kind of future storms were ahead.

Besides, the likelihood of me meeting anyone interesting was slim to none, considering I rarely left the condo. And that was fine with me. I tend to fall into relationships like mud puddles. I'll be strolling along, minding my own business, and the next thing I know, I'm ten years into a long-term, committed relationship without even realizing what happened.

Sure, relationships are fun, but they can also be some of the most painful experiences on earth. I wasn't anywhere nearly recovered from my last relationship to even entertain the idea of falling into another one.

For the moment, my plan was to simply enjoy my life untethered.

# The Kiss

After cocktails, we hopped on the beach trolley and headed down to the strip, a stretch of restaurants and shops along Clearwater Beach. After hitting a few of the touristy hot spots and watching the sunset, we came to a crosswalk, where I noticed two people with clipboards on the opposite side of the street.

"What do you think is on those clipboards?" I asked my friend.

"Well, there's only one way to find out," she said, pulling my sleeve and dragging me across the street.

We approached the people holding the mysterious clipboards, and I launched into my inquisition. What kinds of questions are you asking? Are you a non-profit? What are you going to do with the information you gather here?

What can I say? I've always been a curious soul, and I have questions about everything.

And that's when I heard a voice behind me. "Where y'all from?"

It was a man's voice. I assumed my friend would handle that conversation, since I was clearly busy with the clipboards.

Eventually, the surveyors grew tired of my questions and I was forced to turn back to my friend, who was now deep into a conversation with the stranger.

"How about you. Where are you from?" he asked me.

"I grew up here, but now I'm a gypsy," I said.

"Where did you go to school?" he asked.

"Largo," I said.

"Me too!" he said.

With that recognition, my friend grabbed the stranger by the arm and said, "You're coming with us." He didn't resist.

We walked to a nearby bar and ordered some drinks. And in a matter of minutes, I learned that his name was Shawn, and that we'd attended the same high school for a short time during the same time period, but had never met each other. I stared at him trying to envision what he might have looked like then, and whether we might have ever passed by each other in the hall.

Several drinks and another bar later, the words I spoke to Tawnya earlier on the balcony seemed to no longer apply. Seven months after I sat on a brown couch thinking that I'd never find happiness again, much less feel anything again, there I was, kissing a random stranger that my friend pulled off the street.

Maybe it was the fact that we'd gone to the same high school together. Maybe it was because the conversation with him was so easy. Maybe it was the cocktails. Or, maybe it was that I was more ready than I realized to feel something again. Because I couldn't deny that I did, indeed, feel something.

It was reassuring to know that all the grieving hadn't numbed my heart permanently. As the night faded into the wee hours of the morning, we exchanged phone numbers and Tawnya and I headed back to the condo.

As I drifted off to sleep, I felt grateful to finally feel alive again. And I was grateful that I'd had the courage to go.

*- THE END -*

# -Afterword-

There were seven months of deep, spiritual growth between the conversation on the couch and the conversation in the bar. One ending, and one beginning.

Looking back, I still can't believe how perfectly orchestrated the timing of everything was. Every experience arrived right on time. Every teacher and every lesson showed up when I was ready to learn. And that's when I realized that everything that happens in life generally happens at exactly the right time.

The Trip:
4/22/18 – Conversation on the couch
4/30/18 – Said goodbye to Zoey
5/8/18 – Lost the white Sprinter van
5/9/18 – Bought the gray Sprinter van
5/10/18 – Filed for divorce
5/11/18 – Put the house on the market
5/15/18 – Sold the house
5/18/18 – Picked up my gray Sprinter van
6/8/18 – Closed on the house
7/4/18 – Left on my cross-country trip
7/28/18 – Manifested the beach condo
8/13/18 – Finalized my divorce
11/18/18 – Conversation in the bar

In those seven months, I experienced the adventure of a lifetime. I could have chosen a million different paths after that life-changing conversation on the couch. But I chose the one that was filled with adventure.

But my lifestyle redesign didn't happen in a single moment.

It happened over several cups of coffee while reading books like *No Mud, No Lotus, The Gifts of Imperfection, Man's Search for Meaning*, and *A Course in Miracles*.

It happened at a number of state parks and national forests across the U.S., where my problems felt insignificant next to the expansive beauty of nature.

It happened during a 2-hour massage, where I felt the unconditional love and support from a woman whose compassionate spirit I will never forget.

It happened at Lake Sammamish, while staring up at four bald eagles circling above me, reminding me of my freedom, strength, and independence.

It happened in the Mojave Desert, while I drove for hours in silence with nothing but my thoughts.

It happened at the Grand Canyon, where my sorrow faded further into the dark depths of the gorge.

It happened in Austin, TX, while surrounded by the laughter of old friends.

And it happened on Clearwater Beach, where the warm air somehow also revived my heart.

After traveling more than 10,000 miles across the country in my van, I spent four months in a condo on the beach. And in that time, I completely redesigned my life. The adventure gave me the time and space to grieve the loss of my marriage, and accept that my life will never look exactly the way I think it will. And that's okay.

Today, without the burden of my heavy secret, I'm more open to seeing life's messy moments differently. I have more compassion for those who have been where I've been. And it feels good to no longer hold negative energy about the people or the circumstances that led to my suffering.

I'm finally able to see that everything happened for me, rather than to me.

And I see now that my choice to leave—to go—wasn't so much about running away from the painful memories as it was about running toward my future. Because the truth is, you won't know you're ready until you're ready. But when you're ready, you'll go.

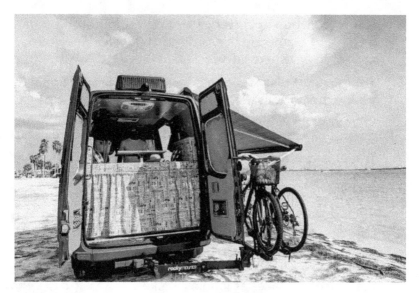

*The van on the beach*

*Here are some of my greatest takeaways from that trip:*

1. **You get to choose how you respond to everything.** You may not get to choose how your life unfolds, but you do get to choose if and how you respond to everything that happens. Life is full of change, but it's also full of choices.

2. **No matter what happens, everything's going to be okay.** While it might not seem like it in the moment, everything is going to be okay...eventually.

3. **If you don't own it, you can't change it.** Whenever a relationship ends—whether it's a friendship or an intimate partnership—it's essential that you understand your role in it. Until you're able to stop blaming someone else for your problems, and start taking responsibility for your own happiness, the negative energy will steal your joy.

4. **Boundaries are nothing if you don't honor them.** If you don't clearly define and communicate your boundaries— what you will and will not accept from other people—you can rest assured, your boundaries will be crossed, leaving you feeling taken advantage of.

5. **Roots can be replanted.** Planting roots doesn't mean they'll stay planted in the same place forever. They can be replanted anywhere, at any time.

6. **Your level of disappointment is directly proportional to your expectations.** People can only ever fail your expectations of them. When you experience a big disappointment, check your expectations. It's possible they were unrealistic.

7. **Travel is good medicine.** Never underestimate the value of a change of pace and a change of scenery. Travel is therapeutic, offering small doses of humility, perspective, and gratitude.

8. **Grieving takes as long as it takes.** There are no hard and fast rules when it comes to grieving. For some people, grieving takes months, and for others, it takes years. Don't rush the process. It takes as long as it takes.

9. **If you don't ask, you don't get.** If you want something, ask for it. Because the answer will always be 'no' until you ask. There are infinite possibilities waiting for you, so keep asking.

10. **If someone wants to leave your life, let them.** Allow people to come in and out of your life without manipulation or resistance. Those who want to be in your life will stay; those who don't will go. And that's a good thing.

11. **Go where you are led.** Trust your intuition to lead you where you are supposed to go. Anything else is just overcomplicating things.

12. **Impermanence is a sure thing.** Nothing, and I do mean nothing, lasts forever. Everything in the natural world is in a constant state of change. We are constantly growing and evolving, and embracing that reality that change is inevitable makes it easier to accept when it arrives.

13. **Love attracts love.** What you give is what you get. Like attracts like, and love attracts love. And when you withhold love—as a form of punishment or as a demand for love— you are also withholding love from yourself.

14. **Self-care is powerful.** By building a strong self-care foundation, you'll create the conditions for ease, health, self-confidence, strength, and resilience.

15. **Everyone is a teacher.** Every person who shows up in your life is there to teach you something. Pay attention.

16. **Allow all emotions.** Suppressing your emotions will only intensify them. Allow all of your emotions to flow freely, so they can move through you more quickly.

17. **Stop giving a damn what other people think of you.** One of my favorite Eleanor Roosevelt quotes is this one: "What other people think of me is none of my business." And it's so true. Most opinions have more to do with the opinion-holder than anyone else. You're better off being so busy living your life that you don't even notice or care what others think of you.

18. **Everything in life happens at exactly the right time.** Every life experience happens exactly as it should, and at exactly the right time. It's just that most of the time it doesn't make sense until much later.

19. **You'll remember it differently.** Time really does alter your perceptions and memories. Over time, you'll see your experiences differently.

20. **Stay open.** While it's important to have goals and a clear vision of the life you want to experience, staying open is vital. Once you get clear on what you want, be sure to stay open to how it all unfolds.

21. **Life is easy.** Life can be hard, or it can be easy. That's a choice only you can make for yourself.

22. **You are stronger than you think you are.** When you need the strength to push through a seemingly impossible situation, you'll find it. You are much stronger than you think.

23. **Forgiveness is a process.** Forgiveness isn't meant to simply be understood conceptually; it's meant to be experienced. Forgiveness is a habit. It's something you learn to do again and again. It isn't about forgetting or ignoring that something painful happened. It's simply a process of realizing

there is nothing to forgive. And because I now understand that, I would willingly re-experience all of this again if given the choice.

24. **Life's too short to live a shitty one.** Use the good china. Drink the good wine. Go on more adventures. Start working on your bucket list right now…and stop saving all the good stuff for later.

# - Acknowledgments -

So many beautiful souls have supported me through this incredible life-changing journey. I will be forever grateful for your friendship, encouragement, and support.

To my creator, for giving me the greatest gift of all: life. It has been such an amazing journey thus far, and I feel blessed to have experienced so many wonderful lessons and adventures.

To my parents, for supporting all of my crazy, unconventional dreams. Thank you for teaching me the importance of humor, creativity, and love.

To Jaime Highfield, for the beautiful cover and interior design work on this book, as well as many other projects. I'm grateful for your friendship, patience, and attention to detail. (Instagram: @designstudiofortyeight)

To Val Serdy and Bethany Petersen for your valuable input on the content and organization of this book. Thank you for helping me make the story better. (Instagram: @bethanyapetersen)

To Lisa Fischer, for helping me recover my sense of self-confidence and self-worth. Our work together has been nothing short of life changing. "Champagne and Chickens" still makes me smile every time. (www.lisafischerstyling.com)

To Brenda Reiss, for your graceful presence, gentle inquiry, and loving guidance as I navigated the transformational forgiveness process. (www.brendareisscoaching.com)

And to my readers—the dreamers of the world who, like me, are refusing to save all the good stuff for later. Cheers to squeezing life's giant lemon and to going on lots of soul-filling adventures.

XOXO
Stacy

## ABOUT THE AUTHOR

# Stacy Fisher

**STACY FISHER** is a registered dietitian, lifestyle coach, health & travel writer, and speaker with more than 20 years of experience in the healthcare industry. As the founder of LivingUpp, she teaches women how to build a solid self-care foundation using a unique framework and planning system that she developed. Her methodology empowers women to simplify their lifestyles, so they can experience more ease and better health. Stacy has been featured in *The Costco Connection* and is the author of three other books, including *The Lifestyle Design Planner*.

### www.LivingUpp.com

**Coaching.** Work with Stacy to redesign your lifestyle and create more ease and better health.

**Speaking.** Book Stacy to speak at an upcoming conference, workshop, or team meeting.

**Writing.** Hire Stacy to help with a special writing project.

▶ StacyFisher

⊙ @livingupp

f LivingUppdates

𝓟 @livingupp

in Stacy Fisher

✉ Share@LivingUpp.com

🌐 www.LivingUpp.com